Occupational Wellbeing

Edited by Kavitha Palaniappan and Pamela McCauley

Published in London, United Kingdom

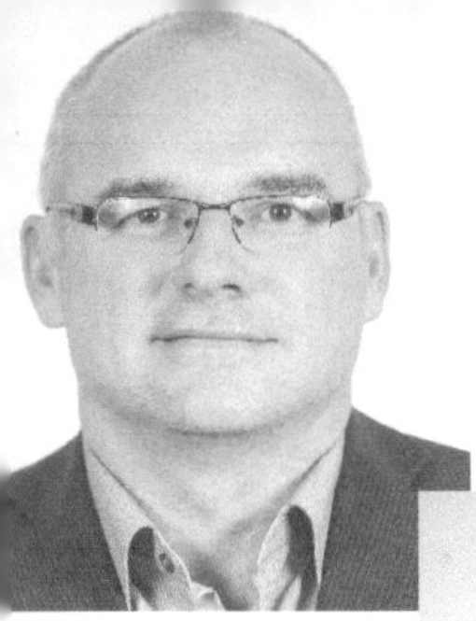
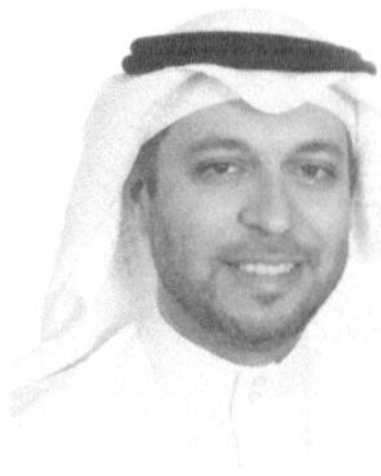
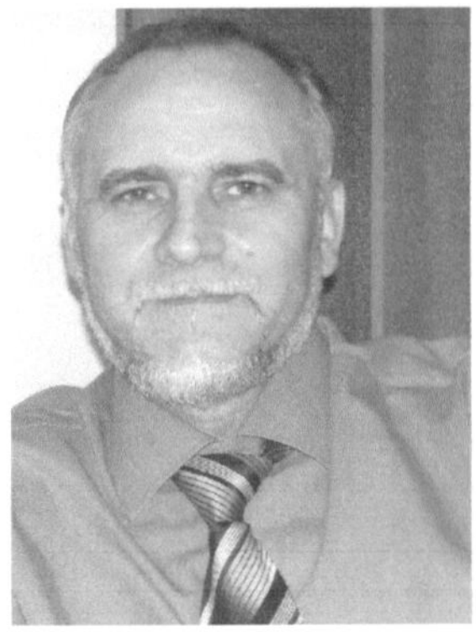
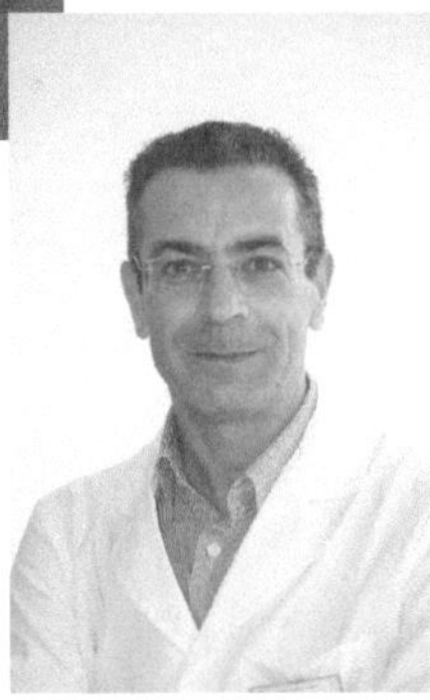
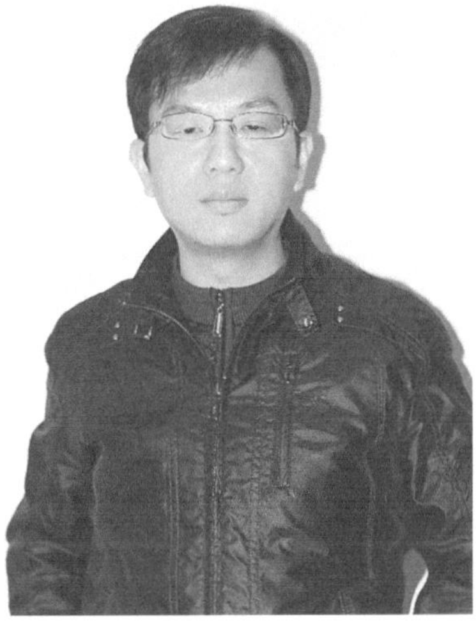
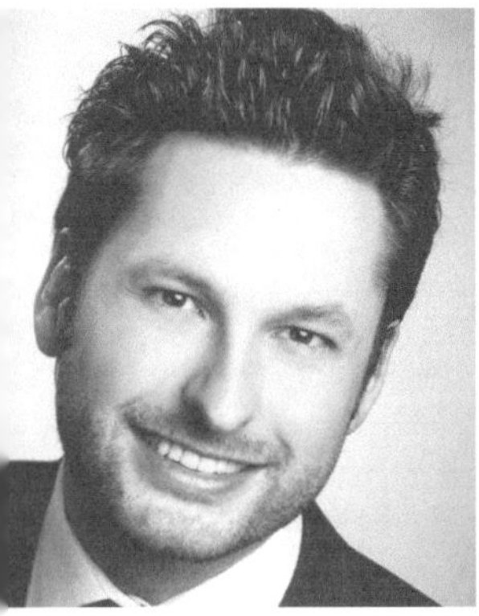
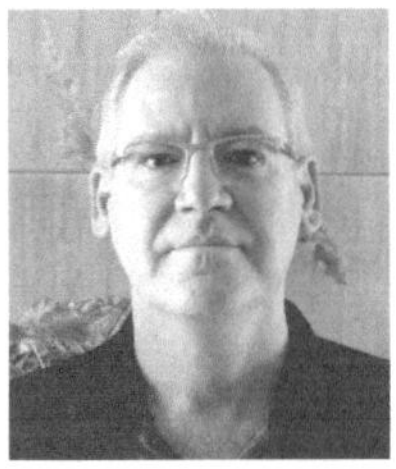

IntechOpen

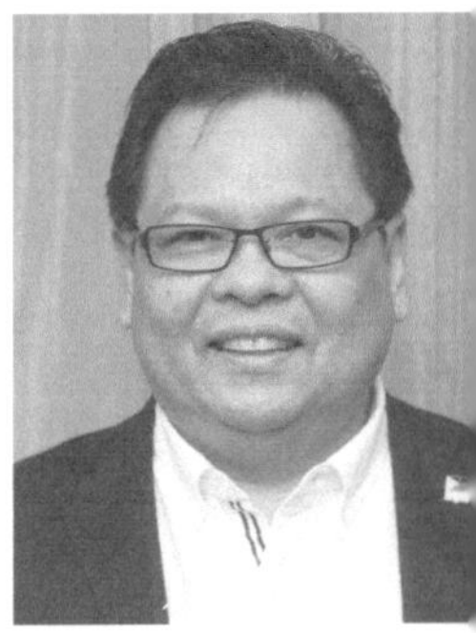
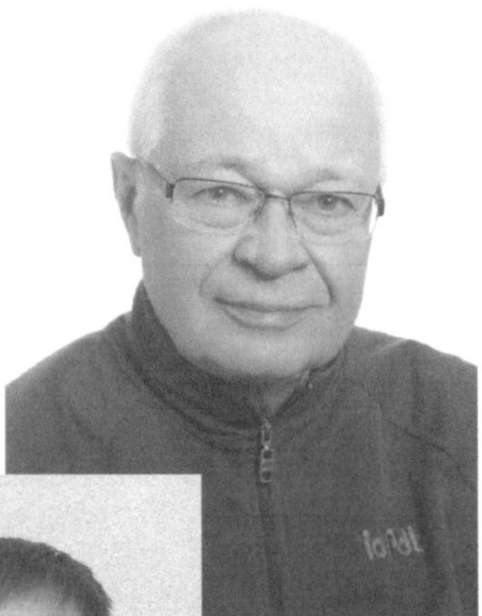
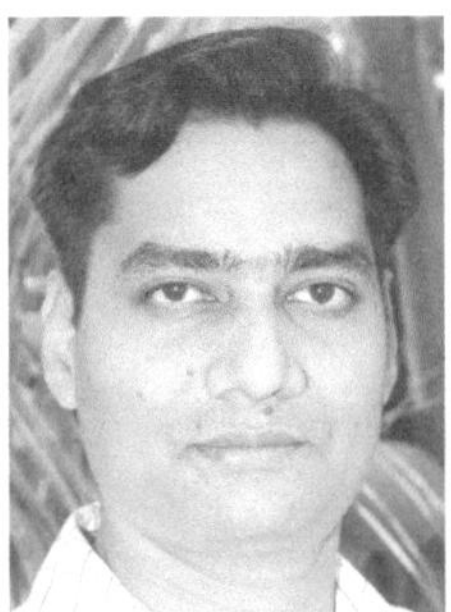
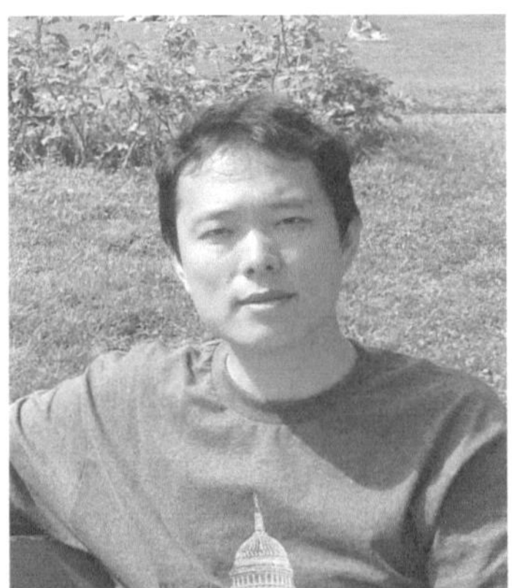
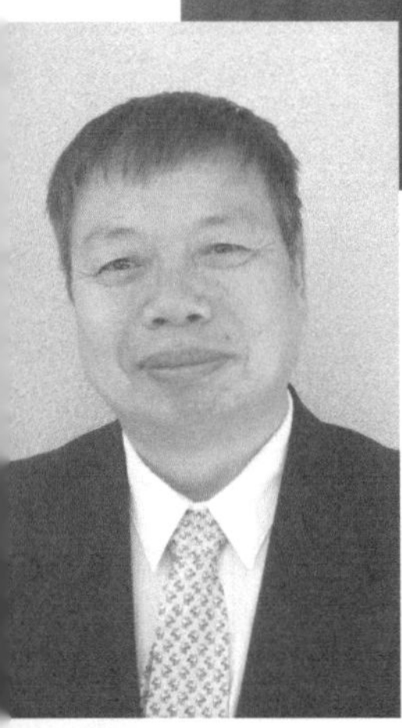
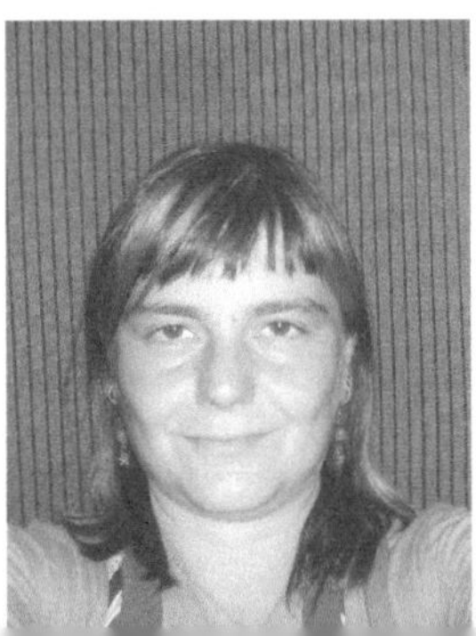

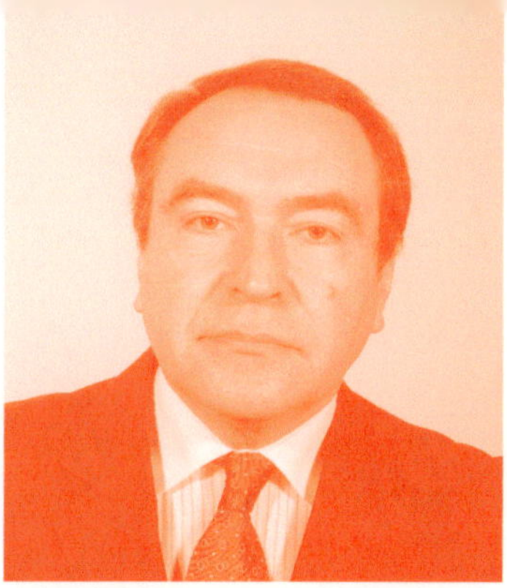
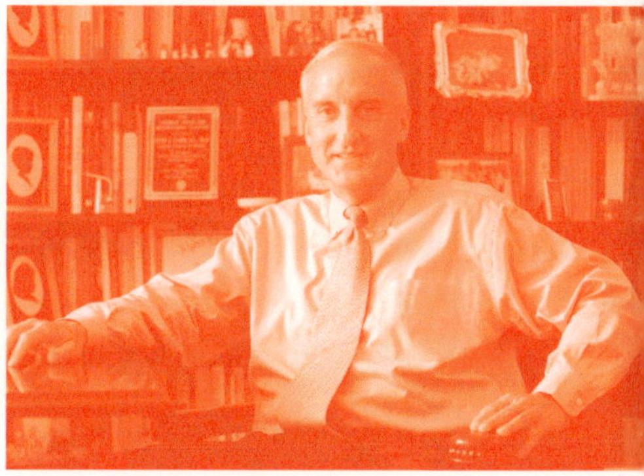
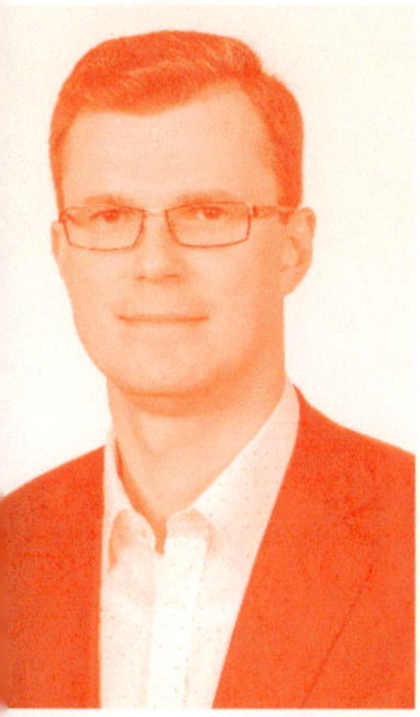
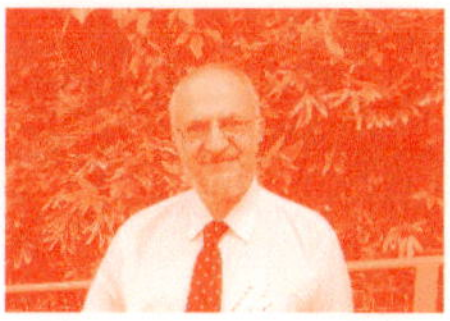
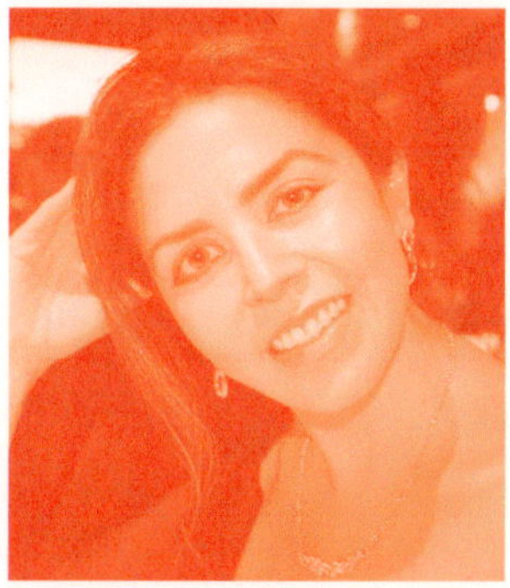

Supporting open minds since 2005

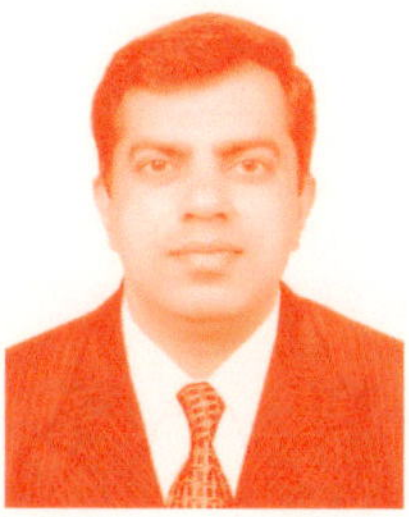
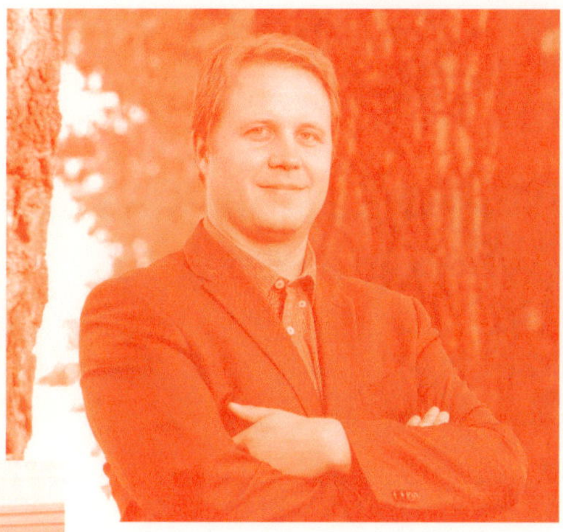
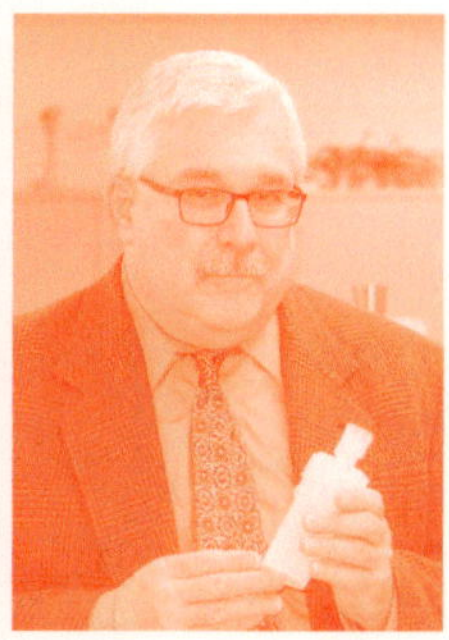
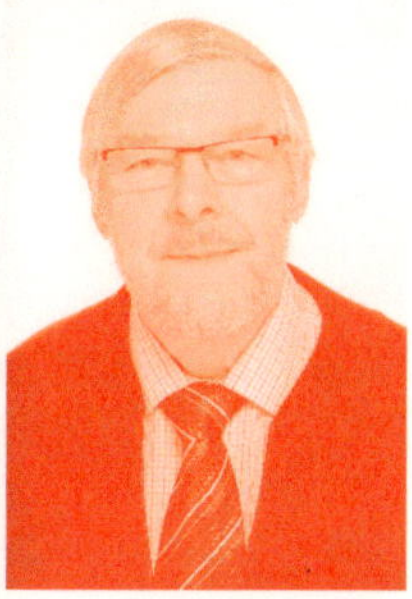
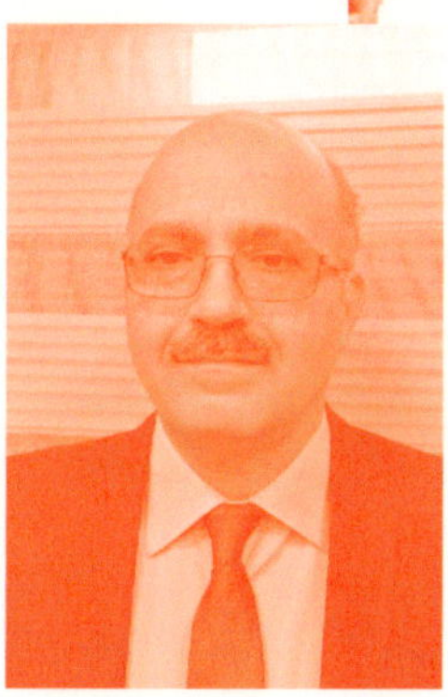
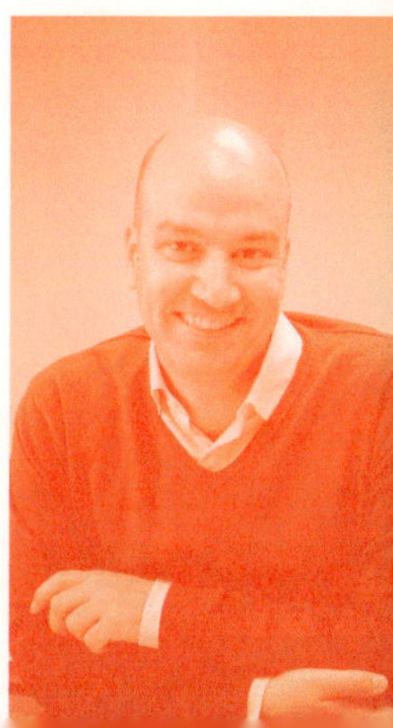
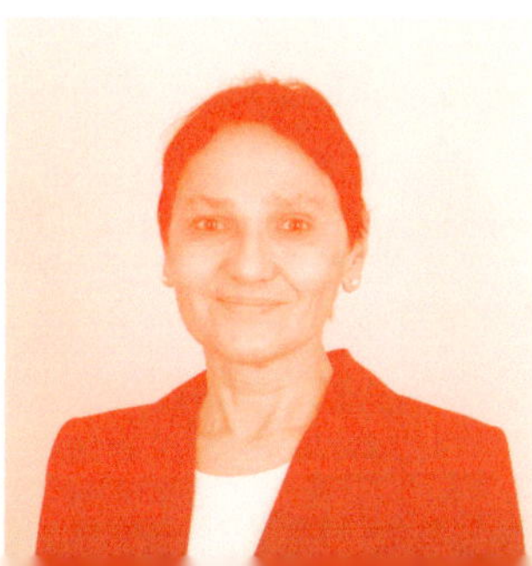

Occupational Wellbeing
http://dx.doi.org/10.5772/intechopen.87327
Edited by Kavitha Palaniappan and Pamela McCauley

Assistant to the Editor: Anthony Dixon

Contributors
Ömer Alkan, Sena Gültekin, Swarna Weerasinghe, Gyan Kashyap, Praveen Chokhandre, Shri Kant Singh, Krishnan Srinivasan, Smisha Mohan, Jeneth Berlin Raj T, Wahab Gbenga Ojebiyi, Olalekan Olaoye, Irtyah Merchaoui, Ines Rassas, Nidhal Mlik, Mhenni Feten, Imen Miled, Charfeddine Amri, Marouen Hayouni, Thomas Gilliam, Paul Terpeluk, Ozlem Koseoglu Ornek, Nurcan Kolaç, Judith P. Andersen, Jennifer F. Chan, Chiraz Guedda, Amira Omrane, Taoufik Khalfallah, Lamia Bouzgarrou, Surya Pratap Singh Somvanshi, Surendra Prasad Tripathi, Srk Singh, Anupam Mishra, Priyadarshini Dasgupta

First published in London, United Kingdom, 2021 by IntechOpen
IntechOpen is the global imprint of INTECHOPEN LIMITED, registered in England and Wales, registration number: 11086078, 5 Princes Gate Court, London, SW7 2QJ, United Kingdom
Printed in Croatia

British Library Cataloguing-in-Publication Data
A catalogue record for this book is available from the British Library

Additional hard and PDF copies can be obtained from orders@intechopen.com

Occupational Wellbeing
Edited by Kavitha Palaniappan and Pamela McCauley
p. cm.
Print ISBN 978-1-83962-338-7
Online ISBN 978-1-83962-339-4
eBook (PDF) ISBN 978-1-83962-340-0

Meet the editor

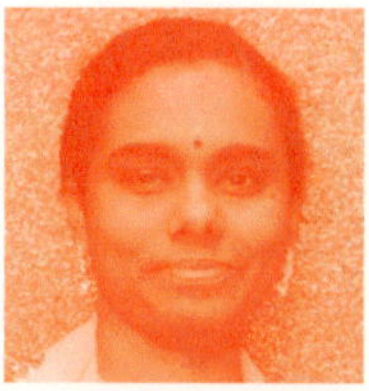

Associate Professor Dr. Kavitha Palaniappan is the academic director at Newcastle Australia Institute of Higher Education, a wholly-owned entity of the University of Newcastle, Australia. She teaches the program of Bachelor of Environmental and Occupational Health and Safety (BEnvOHS). Apart from teaching, Dr. Palaniappan is also actively involved in multi-disciplinary research, including the prevalence of psychosocial illnesses and their impacts on society, economy and country. She also researches alternative therapies to enhance sleep, yoga and its health benefits, the toxicity of nanomaterials, exposure measurements and hygiene requirements for nano-titanium dioxide, exposure to nano-silver in mattresses and beddings and their health effects, associations between seasonal patterns, climate variables, and dengue risks in Singapore. She is a graduate member of the Institution of Occupational Safety and Health (IOSH).

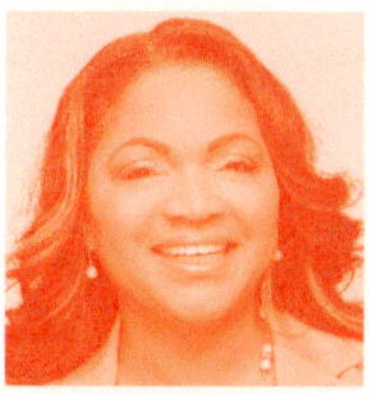

Dr. Pamela McCauley is Associate Dean for Academic Programs, Diversity, Equity, and Inclusion in the Wilson College of Textiles, North Carolina State University. She is an internationally recognized industrial engineering researcher in the development of mathematical models, ergonomics, biomechanics, and leadership in STEM. Dr. McCauley served as the director of the Ergonomics Laboratory in the Department of Industrial Engineering, University of Central Florida, and as the program director for the National Science Foundation, Computer Information Science and Engineering Directorate's I-Corps Program. She previously held the position of Martin Luther King, Jr. Visiting Associate Professor of Aeronautics and Astronautics at the Massachusetts Institute of Technology (MIT). She has written more than 100 technical publications, an internationally used ergonomics textbook, and books on STEM leadership.

Contents

Preface **XI**

Section 1
Sectorial Analysis of Occupational Health and Safety **1**

Chapter 1 **3**
The Importance of Exposure Assessment in Blue Collar Jobs: Construction as an Example
by Priyadarshini Dasgupta

Chapter 2 **15**
Occupational Health Hazards Associated with Nigerian Fisheries
by Olalekan Jacob Olaoye and Wahab Gbenga Ojebiyi

Chapter 3 **33**
Occupational Health and Safety Standards of Foreign Seasonal Farm Workers: Evaluation of Personal Protection Measures, Policies and Practices
by Swarna Weerasinghe

Chapter 4 **53**
A Review of Ergonomic Evaluation of Occupational Hazard of Indian Agriculture Farm and Allied Activities
by Surendra Prasad Tripathi, Surya Pratap Singh Somvanshi, Shyam Ranjan Kumar Singh and Anupam Mishra

Chapter 5 **67**
Ergonomic Evaluation of Thermal Stress in a Tunisian Steel Industry
by Amira Omrane, Taoufik Khalfallah and Lamia Bouzgarrou

Chapter 6 **77**
Responsiveness of Occupational Health Risk and Preventive Measures Practice by the Workers Employed in Tannery Occupation in Kanpur, India
by Gyan Chandra Kashyap, Praveen Chokhandre and Shri Kant Singh

Section 2
Physiological and Psychosocial Wellbeing **95**

Chapter 7 **97**
Muscle Health: The Gateway to Population Health Management
by Thomas Gilliam and Paul Terpeluk

Chapter 8 115
Physiological Stress Responses Associated with High-Risk Occupational Duties
by Jennifer F. Chan and Judith P. Andersen

Chapter 9 131
Modeling the Factors That Affect Work Accidents with Binary Logistic Regression: Evidence from Turkey
by Ömer Alkan and Sena Gültekin

Chapter 10 147
Occupational Heat Stress: A Technical Scan
by Krishnan Srinivasan, Smisha Mohan and Jeneth Berlin Raj T

Chapter 11 159
Managing Inter-Organizational Knowledge Sharing: Integrating Macro, Meso and Micro Level Analysis
by Chiraz Guedda

Chapter 12 175
Quality of Life in Employee with Workaholism
by Ozlem Koseoglu Ornek and Nurcan Kolac

Chapter 13 191
Influence of Tunisian Revolution on Bullying at Work in Interns and Residents
by Irtyah Merchaoui, Ines Rassas, Marouen Hayouni, Nidhal Mlik, Feten Mhenni, Imen Miled and Charfeddine Amri

Preface

Although many books address the concept of "health," there is still a need for in-depth analysis of aspects of health associated with various occupations and their impacts on society and the economy. This book, *Occupational Wellbeing*, examines the risks for various diseases in a range of workplace environments.

This book is divided into two sections. Section 1 analyses the occupational health and safety parameters in various occupational sectors such as the construction industry, fisheries, agriculture industry, steel industry, and tanneries. Section 2 focuses on physiological and psychosocial wellbeing.

The construction industry is an industry that mostly employs migrant workers from many countries, as the local population is not usually keen to take up those jobs. Hence, the occupational health and safety of these migrant workers are not usually a priority compared to the local population. Hence, Chapter 1 addresses the need to cater to these workers' wellbeing.

Chapter 2 explores the occupational issues experienced by the various value chain actors in the fisheries industry, be it artisanal fishery or aquaculture, or industry fishery. Chapter 3 reviews the legislative framework that is in place to safeguard the occupational health and safety of foreign seasonal farm workers, whereas Chapter 4 evaluates the ergonomic hazards of Indian agriculture farms and allied activities. Moving along the same concept of ergonomic evaluation, Chapter 5 analyses the impact of thermal stress in the steel industry. The last chapter in Section 1 explores the extent of awareness of occupational health and safety in the tannery industry.

The second section of the book begins with a chapter on the importance of skeletal muscle followed by a chapter about how the body responds physiologically to high-risk occupational duties. Chapter 9 figures out the factors that could potentially be associated to typical work accidents. Chapter 10 presents a technical scan of occupational heat stress and its impacts on the workers. Chapter 11 brings out the importance of inter-organizational knowledge to develop an integrative occupational health and safety model. The last two chapters in this section are dedicated to psychosocial wellbeing and review the quality of life of people deemed to be "workaholics." The final chapter examines bullying in the workplace.

This book gives an overall picture of the current occupational health scenario, and I trust readers will enjoy the intensity of scientific data and the depth of analysis in each of the chapters. I wish you all a happy reading experience.

Best Wishes!

Kavitha Palaniappan
Newcastle Australia Institute of Higher Education,
(a wholly owned entity of The University of Newcastle, Australia),
Singapore

Pamela McCauley
Wilson College of Textiles,
North Carolina State University,
Raleigh, North Carolina, United States of America

Section 1

Sectorial Analysis of Occupational Health and Safety

Chapter 1

The Importance of Exposure Assessment in Blue Collar Jobs: Construction as an Example

Priyadarshini Dasgupta

Abstract

Exposure to musculoskeletal disorder (MSDs) risk factors are not only common but also omnipresent in almost every workplace. The purpose of this chapter is to describe how we can attempt to reduce the exposure to the risk factor in order to attain a reduction in negative physiological outcomes (like injuries and illnesses). Blue collar jobs are often subject to heavy manual handling and intervening these jobs with any new technique is burdensome. This chapter gives the example of construction job as a blue collar and hard to reach job in which an intervention was implemented in a systematic way.

Keywords: construction, intervention, exposure, physical, ceiling, installation, hazards

1. Introduction

The construction sector is dynamic and usually follows a rigid work schedule. The high number of acute and chronic injuries and illnesses put construction sector as one of the most dangerous workplaces in the United States. Due to the production-oriented nature of the job, exposure to the risk factors is not uncommon in construction related jobs. Opportunity of using the personal protective equipment (PPEs) is not scarce but high production pressure necessitates the workers to focus more on the outcome than a safe procedure.

The author of this chapter has carried out several focus groups in different construction sectors in greater Boston area. In the author's experience, the workers most of the time, discussed on the issues of the weight of the panels. It is noteworthy that in any focus groups, the workers did not participate well if the facilitator used words like 'safety', 'problem', 'research' or 'solution'. However, the workers spontaneously participated while they were asked about 'any concern they can share' with the facilitator. In such focus groups, the workers were supposed to brainstorm with any possible ideas of implementing or using an assistive device for ceiling installation. Before we learn about the possible solutions, let us have a look at the problems associated with ceiling installation in the following.

2. Drywall panel installation

The main operation of drywall carpentry is installation of the drywall panels onto the walls and ceilings. Installation of drywall panels is faster and cheaper than plaster walls. The drywall installers lay out the whole interior wall system and ceiling with studs and hang large drywall panels to the ceiling and sidewalls.

Drywall panels consist of a layer of gypsum (often used as building material) between two layers of heavy paper. In commercial applications, the standard sizes are 4 ft. X 8 ft. and 4 ft. X 12 ft. with a 5/8 inch thickness. The usual weight of a 4 ft. X 8 ft. panel is 70 lbs. and that of a 4 ft. X 12 ft. is 105 lb. [1]. The panels used in residential carpentry are 4 ft. X 8 ft. with a thickness of ½ inch.

The main difference between residential and commercial drywall installation is the use of wood studs in residential carpentry instead of lighter metal studs in commercial carpentry. As far as the hanging of the drywall itself is concerned, there are no other significant differences between the two settings.

In the case of ceiling installation, usually a pair of installers lifts the panels to the ceiling while standing on separate ladders. One of the installers continues to hold the panel to the ceiling while the other installer uses the screw gun and affixes the panel permanently on his side. The first installer then releases one of his hands to use the screw gun until the panel becomes attached to the ceiling (**Figure 1**). In the case of smaller drywall pieces, one installer instead of two carries out the process.

For wall installation, the entire 4 ft. X 8 ft. or 4 ft. X 12′ pieces are attached vertically to the wall; this is often carried out by a single installer. For walls more than 12′ high, wall installation might include horizontal attachment of more than one panel.

The main tasks of the drywall installation process, which the workers carry out in a routine sequential order, are as follows [2]:

- **Stacking:** After getting unloaded from the truck, the drywall panels are stacked at the site on different floors. Generally the panels are put on each floor by a crane and then pulled through the window of the respective floors. In absence of an elevator, the workers carry the drywall panels through the stairs.

- **Carrying:** Carrying is required to bring the panels from the place of stacking to the place of installation. Workers also need to carry the panels for housekeeping and fitting (both described below).

- **Measuring:** The panels are measured according to the dimensions needed. This is done before cutting and installing them in the desired place.

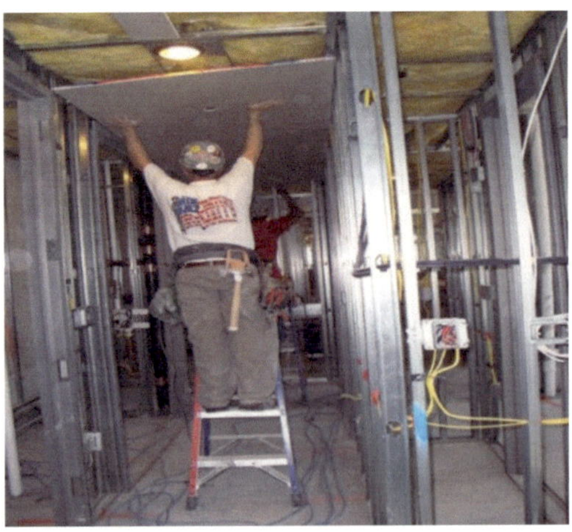

Figure 1.
Holding the panel, being on ladder.

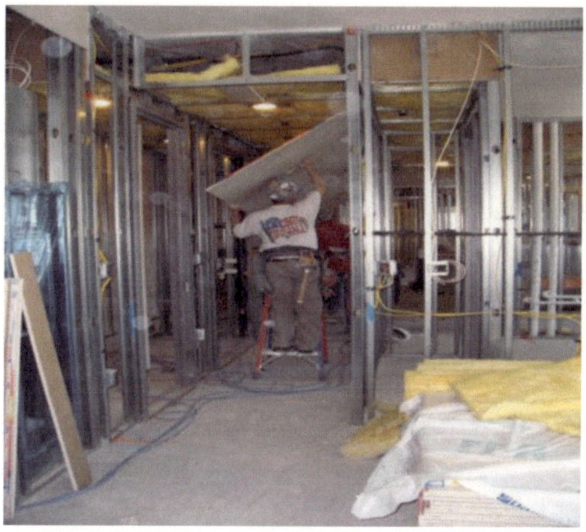

Figure 2.
Lifting the panel.

- **Cutting:** The panels are cut into the necessary dimensions. There are two main cutting operations: a) cutting of whole panels into two or more pieces, b) selective cutting of smaller parts to fit them around doors, windows, electrical and plumbing outlets.

- **Fitting:** Cut panels are measured several times before installing them.

- **Lifting:** In the case of lifting the panels to the ceiling, the workers might stand on a ladder or scissor lift based on the height of the wall, as shown in **Figure 2**.

- **Attaching:** Attachment of the panels is done with a screw gun. In case of attachment to the ceiling, workers might work in pairs. One of them holds the panel while the other one screws it into the studs (**Figure 1**).

- **Housekeeping:** At the end of a work day, the workers remove rejected pieces to the trash and keep the unused pieces back at designated places for the next day's use.

3. Handling and carrying heavy drywall panels as sources of exposure

Handling and carrying the heavy and bulky drywall panels have been cited as exposure sources for the high amount of back and shoulder muscle injuries of drywall carpenters. Handling of heavy drywall pieces was reported by [3], to be associated with more than 40 percent of the overexertion injuries of drywall workers. In this study, more than 15% of total traumatic injuries were muscle overexertion due to lifting of the heavy drywall panels, whereas 37.2% of total traumatic injuries were injuries due to bodily reaction while handling the drywall panels.

4. Biomechanical stress exerted on back when lifting panels as a source of exposure

Ref. [4] analyzed the four most common techniques (three horizontal and one vertical) used to lift a drywall panel and showed that each lifting technique exerted a minimum of 655 lb. disc compression force on the low back (L5/S1 region) of the workers whether for a 60 lb., 80 lb. or 100 lb. drywall panel. The same study found that low back loading while lifting a 100 lb. drywall panel exceeds 760 lb., the maximum value recommended by NIOSH in the Work Practices Guide for Manual Lifting. All four lifting techniques also involved risk of perturbation in postural balance [5].

Yuan et. Al., [2] found that the average disc compression force during installation of drywall panels exceeded value of 760 lb. (3400 N) disc compression force, set by NIOSH as the recommended action limit. The highest value of disc compression force in this study was found to be 1721 lb. (7748.8 N) and was sustained for an average of 8.5% of the total 8 hour work shift, or around 41 minutes.

5. PATH (posture, activities, tools, and handling) data collection

PATH method [6, 7], was used to code posture, activities, tools used and materials handled at every moment for at least 3–4 hours every day with a hierarchical taxonomy. Since the drywall installation task is cyclical in nature, we collected data for a week that is absolutely representative of the whole task. We used fixed intervals to make direct observations and coded postures into a PDA.

6. 3DSSPP (three dimensional static strength prediction program)

3DSSPP (3 Dimensional Static Strength Prediction Program) was utilized in order to find out the compressive forces generated at low back and shoulder moments generated in the ceiling installers.

The sequence of static postures was selected while performing the task of ceiling drywall installation. The selected static postures from the task videos were not made at a defined interval of seconds or minutes. Instead, the postures were selected corresponding to the main set of activities. For example, the task of installing the drywall to the ceiling at the intervention phase comprised the following six activities, i) loading the panels to the electrical lift, ii) lifting the panels while being on the lift, iii) raising the panels to the ceiling, iv) holding the panels to the ceiling, v) attaching the panes to the ceiling.

7. Research design

This intervention study was designed as a quasi-experimental study with no control group. The only experimental group consisted of the five drywall installers.

Baseline PHASE	Intervention PHASE
Static frame description	
Lifting the drywall in overhead arm posture	Sliding the drywall panel to the electrical lift, both arms down
Carrying the drywall panel in overhead arm posture and stepping on the ladder	Keeping the hands on the drywall panel being raise by the electrical lift
One feet in air, maintaining the previous posture	The arms are down, maintaining the previous posture
Holding the drywall panel (overhead arms) to the ceiling, drywall in air	Overhead arms, drywall being lifted to the ceiling and supported by 'deadman'

Table 1.
The selected static frames from the videos for 3DSSPP analysis.

To find out a change of exposure **for ceiling installation at the intervention phase compared to the baseline phase**, a before- after comparison protocol (for PATH and 3DSSPP) was followed.

Table 1 summarizes the overall description of the main postural activities which were selected as the static frames for baseline and intervention analysis in 3DSSPP method.

8. Prior ergonomic interventions in drywall installation that was discussed with the installers

As mentioned earlier, the idea of having the focus groups was to engage the workers to brainstorming sessions in order to find out a solution to their concerns of ceiling/sidewall installation. Some of the ideas that the facilitator of those focus groups brought to the discussion are as follows:

A. Coupling devices for carrying the panel were already introduced by [8] in order to reduce awkward trunk postures while carrying the drywall panels. Installers were of the opinion that the coupling tools would be suitable for carrying, but could not be used as a help during installation of the panels simply because they lost time for removing the coupling tools from the panel before the installation process.

B. Although stilts have not been tested as an alternative to the ladders for drywall installers, workers tend to put extra efforts on their lower extremity to balance their gait, which results in limiting their joint mobility and increasing the risk for falling over objects [1, 3, 4, 9]. However, a 2009 study by Pan [5] concluded that if stilts are kept at low height, it enables the workers to maintain a good postural balance. The facilitator made it an open question to be answered by the installers.

C. Reducing the weight of drywall panels by cutting it into two pieces would increase the task of fastening additional boards and taping additional joints [1]. The facilitator made it an open question for the installers.

The idea of engaging workers in these focus groups were to receive suggestions from them is a useful way to find a solution for a reduction in exposure(s) [10, 11]. These groups gave the workers an opportunity to speak on their work concerns, to collectively discuss advantages or disadvantages of tools and techniques, and to brainstorm solutions to problems.

8.1 What did the workers suggested from the focus groups

In two different sites, the workers approached the outcome of the focus group quite differently:

a. In site 1, the workers wanted to use a narrow piece of panel that is called a 'deadman' as evidenced by [12].

b. In site B, the workers wanted to give a try with the prototype 'hanger's helper' [13] that was fabricated with the idea of the 'deadman'. We named the prototype 'hanger's helper'.

In both of these sites, the workers took the trial and error method, i.e., they would continue with the devices if they like it and they would stop the trial immediately if they do not like it.

Efficacy studies, usually, are those that proves the accuracy of an instrument or assistive devices to the degree it says it will. By that definition, both 'deadman' and 'hanger's helper' were ready to be assessed for their efficaciousness in the real field. Effectiveness studies, in construction are those that will prove whether any instrument/assistive device would be effective in making a permanent place in the construction trade. This study did not evaluate the effectiveness.

9. The success behind the implementation: some precipitating factors

There were precipitating factors behind the success of implementing the 'deadman' and electrical lift as an intervention. The participants of the intervention or the 'users' had suggested the 'deadman' after perceiving its beneficial use in reducing their overhead arm postures to hold drywall panels to the ceiling. Nevertheless, a brief yet imperative role was played by the safety management crew who gave substantial amount of importance on the safety features of the drywall job at this site. The management was dissatisfied with the potential hazards of the 'bucketing' or 'laddering activities and perceived the electrical lift and 'deadman' to be more stable and therefore safer. The spontaneously yielded to provide one of the two electrical lifts (that were present at the site for some electrical work) for ceiling installation and thus, offered a pivotal support to the 'deadman' use (**Figure 3**).

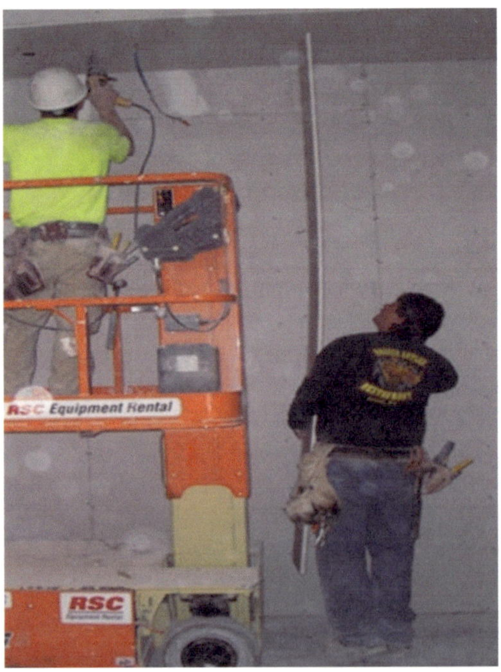

Figure 3.
Use of 'Deadman: narrow piece of panel'.

10. Why exposure assessment is important

The ceiling installation task have many physical exposures that are discussed under sections 3 and 4. These physical exposures are present throughout each cycle in case of a cyclical task or throughout all day (in case it is a non-cyclical task). For example, a ceiling drywall installer will go through the same physical exposures (such as heavy handling, overhead arm postures, back and neck stress) for each ceiling panel installation. Assessment of these exposures will give the opportunity to fix parts of the task. These parts would get fixated by modifying different activities. By doing thus, only a small part of the tasks can get rectified, however, the result oftentimes is a huge reduction in the physical exposure level. If exposure to MSD risk factor is reduced by modifying a task or activity, then usually the modified task or activity gets adopted by all the workers in the organization [14–16]. The next section will describe how and why the exposure was reduced.

11. The reduction in exposure

The physical exposures and risk factors of drywall installation task were handling and holding more than 50 lbs in air with overhead arm postures while being on a ladder and continuously handling and handling such load. The idea of deadman did reduce some part of the exposure such as holding it with overstretched arm posture while raising it towards the ceiling. However, it is noteworthy that the worker standing on the floor still needed to hold the narrow 'deadman' piece with his hand. Deadman is 14 pounds in weight, that is much lighter than the panel weight. As a continuation to this intervention technique, the author was able to implement 'hanger's helper' (**Figure 4**) which was much stable in its base and could be placed on its own to hold the ceiling. These studies were conducted in real field and through the analysis of ergonomic observations at the pre and post intervention phases in real construction workplace settings, evaluated the efficacy of an assistive device for ceiling installation. Detailed analysis of the panel load effect on low back and shoulder joints of the installers were possible due to direct observation of the ceiling installation task at the real construction sites, through video analysis of the task and a clear picture of the shoulder and low back workload of the installers could be drawn. Prior biomechanical studies conducted in simulated laboratory environment did not

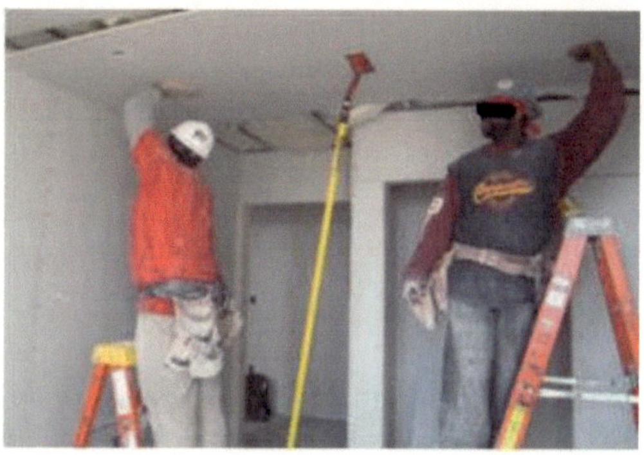

Figure 4.
Use of 'hanger's helper'.

evaluate other biomechanical variables such as shoulder moments while holding the drywall panels to the ceiling, placing the panels to the ceiling, using the neck and head while holding the ceiling or while using the screwgun to attach those panels.

To assess the workers' perception about any reduction in the exposure of ceiling installation, they were anonymously asked questions about their perception on it. Moreover, workers' suggestions on further modification of the tool gave an insight to its future evolution. Hence these exposure assessment methods are an important addition in the long run research on future possibilities on marketing stronger and more stable version of the prototype.

12. The perception of the workers on the interventions

The ceiling installers from the beginning of the study, accepted the idea of participatory research. To them it was something that can simultaneously change their work while they are also doing research. Also, they believed that as a workers' community they could identify what was an important concern, when it became an important concern and what was needed to address the concern. Throughout the installers were of opinion that they loved the interventions, they stated that release of panel loads from their shoulders and neck was the main reason that they liked it. Also, they felt much energetic at work.

13. Summary of the study

The work has examined the physical ergonomic exposures in the ceiling drywall installation task and has established the ergonomic advantage of working with an assistive device during this task. Finding a solution to reduce the exposures in the ceiling installation task was the focus of the study. The initial results were consistent with previous literature that also showed presence of physical exposures such as handling and lifting heavy drywall panels and suggested the high workload as the reason behind the musculoskeletal injury and illness rates of drywall workers. This is the first study that has evaluated the reduction of these exposures of ceiling drywall installation by implementing the ceiling assistive tool as an intervention.

To date, research on drywall carpentry has mostly focused on the workers in simulated working conditions that either analyzed ideal lifting position of the panels or evaluated tools to assist in carrying the panels. This study, through the analysis of ergonomic observations at the on pre and post intervention phases in real construction workplace settings, evaluated the efficacy of an assistive device for ceiling installation and focused on the drywall installers' during real working conditions at the construction fields, which is rare in drywall installation research.

14. Limitations of the study

The main limitation of this dissertation was associated with convenience sampling of sites. As discussed in the introduction section of this dissertation, the difficulty of gaining access to sites did not give much choice other than to focus on a sample of convenience. Thus, the study sites were the only ones tested with the research hypothesis. However, due to high consistency in ceiling installation work, the efficacy results of this study should be reproducible at other sites too.

15. Recommendations for future research

Participatory involvement continues to be a preferred intervention method to reduce the exposure to musculoskeletal risk factors. The workers feel that they are 'empowered' to choose a way of doing the job which makes them more comfortable [17]. This process also makes them able to compare the productivity of the task with the proposed method.

Participatory research can change the lives of the communities as opposed to the academic research. The latter will have a long term effect which can be far away from us. Participatory research has an effect on us while we are doing it. If the research obtains a meaningful data, then an immediate change can be made. The researcher can see the trend and react when community research is obtaining some results and then we can label the change they are having, you can do some permanent changes with it.

Little research on diffusion or adoption of an innovative tool or technique appears to have been conducted in the area of construction intervention. The relative advantage, observability, complexity and compatibility are four of five important criteria that are perceived by the workers in order to decide if an innovation will be adopted by the workers. Despite the explanatory power of perceived attributes, the reason for the scarcity of an investigation might be related to the pre-test phase of an innovation which is kept in confidence for the sake of market research. Future research could bridge this gap by carrying out a thorough qualitative analysis in measuring the five attributes of perception of the relative advantage of an innovation.

Author details

Priyadarshini Dasgupta
Department of Industrial and Engineering Technology, Southeastern Louisiana University, Hammond, Louisiana, USA

*Address all correspondence to: priyadarshini.dasgupta@selu.edu

References

[1] Schneider S., Susi P., 1994. Ergonomics and Construction: A Review of Potential Hazards in New Construction. American Industrial Hygiene Association Journal, 55: 635-649.

[2] Yuan L., Buchholz B., Punnett L., Kriebel D., 2007. Estimation of muscle contraction forces and joint reaction forces at the low back and shoulder during drywall installation. Proceedings of the Human Factors and Ergonomics Society, 2007. 51st Annual Meeting: Baltimore, MD.

[3] Chiou SS., Pan C.S., Bhattacharya A., 2008. Kinematics and kinetics of gait on stilts: identification of risk factors associated with construction stilt use. Ergonomics, 51: 1814-1829.

[4] Pan C.S., Choiu S.S., 1999. Analysis of biomechanical stresses during drywall lifting. International Journal of Industrial Ergonomics, 23:505-511.

[5] Pan C.S., Chiou S., Hendricks S., 2002. The effect of drywall lifting method on workers' balance in a laboratory-based simulation. Occupational Ergonomics. 3: 235-249.

[6] Buchholz B., Paquet V., Punnett L., Lee D., Moir S., 1996. PATH: A work sampling-based approach to Ergonomic job analysis for construction and other on-repetitive work. Applied Ergonomics, 27:177-87.

[7] Moir S., Paquet V., Punnett L., Buchholz B., Wegman D., 2003. Making sense of highway construction: A taxonomic framework for ergonomic exposure assessment and intervention research. Applied Occupational environmental Hygiene, 18(4): 256-267.

[8] Hess J.A., Kincl L.D., Davis K., 2010. The impact of drywall handling tools on the low back. Applied Ergonomics, 41: 305-312.

[9] Pan C.S., Chiou S.S., Hsiao H., Wassell J.T., Keane P.R., 1999. Assessment of perceived traumatic injury hazards during drywall hanging. International Journal of Industrial Ergonomics, 25: 29-37.

[10] Buchholz B., Moir S. and Garrett J., 1999. Health Trak: A participatory approach for ergonomic improvement in construction. In Implementation of Safety and Health on Construction Sites, edited by A Singh, J Hinze and RJ Coble, 711-716, Balkema, Rotterdam.

[11] Buchholz B., Moir S., 1996. Emerging participatory approaches to Ergonomic interventions in the construction industry. American journal of Industrial Medicine, 29: 425-430.

[12] Dasgupta PS., Laura P., Susan M., Sarah K., Buchholz B. Does drywall installers' innovative idea reduce the ergonomic exposures of ceiling installation: a field case study. Applied Ergonomics 2016, 55(July): 183-193.

[13] Dasgupta P., Punnett L., Moir S., Kuhn S., Buchholz B. "Interventions to Reduce the Ergonomic Exposures of Drywall Installation". 6th International Conference on Applied Human Factors and Ergonomics (AHFE 2015) and the Affiliated Conferences, AHFE 2015, Las Vegas, Nevada, USA.

[14] Hess J.A., Hecker S., Weinstein M., Lunger M., 2004. A participatory Ergonomics intervention to reduce risk factors for low-back disorders in concrete laborers. Applied Ergonomics, 35: 427-441.

[15] Kramer D., Bigelow P., Peter V., Garritano E., Carlan N., Wells R., 2009. Spreading good ideas: A case study of the adoption of an innovation in the construction sector. Applied Ergonomics, 40(5): 826-832.

[16] Rempel D., Star D., Barr A., Gibbons B., Janowitz I., 2007. Overhead Drilling: Development and evaluation of a new device. Professional Safety, 52(11): 30-35.

[17] De Jong A.M., Vink P., 2002. Participatory ergonomics applied in installation work. Applied Ergonomics, 33(5):439-48.

Chapter 2

Occupational Health Hazards Associated with Nigerian Fisheries

Olalekan Jacob Olaoye and Wahab Gbenga Ojebiyi

Abstract

Fisheries constitute an important component of Nigeria's agriculture sector contributing meaningfully to the socio-economic development of the nation in terms of employment generation, source of high quality animal protein, and foreign exchange earnings. Despite its significance, fisheries like other agricultural-related activities are not without inherent occupational hazards. The aim of the authors was to review literature on the occupational health hazards associated with the Nigerian fisheries. This was done by specifically reviewing literatures on the linkages between occupational health and sustainable development, overview of occupational hazards, fisheries in Nigeria, and occupational hazards in fisheries with empirical evidences from Nigeria. Based on our review, it was concluded that fisheries like other components of agriculture is a very risky venture which can lead to severe injuries and eventual death if workers' health is not protected and promoted within the industry. It was recommended that occupational health and safety should be promoted within the different value chains of fisheries.

Keywords: aquaculture, fisheries, fish processing, occupational health, occupational hazard, sustainable development

1. Introduction

Nigeria is an oil producing nation. Yet, the nation's economy strongly relies on the agriculture sector. In fact, the nation's economy was described as agrarian before and the first decade after independence. During these periods, the contribution of agriculture was noticed through self-sufficiency from the production of food crops by local farmers making use of crude implements; source of job opportunities especially to unskilled labour in rural areas; exportation of major cash crops such as groundnut, cocoa, kola, etc.; and most importantly meaningful contribution to the country's gross domestic product (GDP). Fisheries, which may be cultured (aquaculture) or captured from either fresh (rivers and lakes) or marine (seas and oceans) water, is one of the subsectors that have been contributing meaningfully to the social and economic development of individuals and the nation at large through agriculture as it serves as the primary means of livelihood to rural dwellers especially those in the riverine areas; and the major source of relatively cheap but quality animal protein in the diets of the people.

Working in the agricultural sector by rural farmers is associated with numerous occupational hazards which were categorized into seven by a combination of authors [1–4] as: (i) Climate: dehydration, heat cramps, heat exhaustion, heat stroke, and skin cancer; (ii) Snakes and insects: injurious bites and stings;

(iii) Tools and farm equipment: Injuries, cuts, and hearing impairment; (iv) Physical labour: musculoskeletal disorders, e.g. pain and fatigue; (v) Pesticides: poisonings, neurotoxicity, reproductive effects, and cancer; (vi) Dusts, fumes, gases, particulates: Irritation, respiratory tract, allergic reactions, respiratory diseases such as asthma, chronic obstructive pulmonary disease, and hypersensitivity pneumonitis, and (vii) Biological agents and vectors of disease: Skin diseases, fungal infections, allergic reactions, malaria, schistosomiasis, sleeping sickness, leishmaniasis, ascariasis, and hookworm.

Work has both social and economic importance because work is done in any society primarily to produce and distribute goods and services that are needed by people in the society [5]. WHO [5] further explains that work plays a psychological role in the formation of self-esteem, a sense of order, and in the shaping of a person's self-identity. Work and sound health are highly and positively correlated in the sense that the more healthy a worker is, the more likely he is to work both effectively and efficiently while an ill-health per positively correlated in the sense that the more healthy a worker is, the more likely he is to work both effectively and efficiently while an ill-health person may likely work effectively and efficiently. Egbetokun [6] reported that a 1% improvement in farmers' health condition will lead to a 21 percent increase in work efficiency. On the other hand, poor farmers' health will reduce income, efficiency and productivity [7]. Hence, for one to work optimally, it is important to keep and maintain sound health especially at the workplace. Like every other work or means of survival and livelihood, the fisheries sector is not without some work-related hazards and risks. In fact, like other agriculture-related works, fisheries have been recognized as one of the riskiest work in the world [8, 9]. Injuries and illnesses are among the health-related factors limiting the productivity from fisheries. According to the Global Burden Disease [10], approximately 2.78 million deaths that occur annually are associated with work-related hazards. The World Health Organization also noted that between 20 and 50 per cents of workers; especially in developing countries like Nigeria are suffering from occupational risks [5].

In Nigeria, fisheries supply and its products come from two broad sources viz. – importation of fish and fisheries products, and local fish production. With the nation's increasing human population, most of whom are youths within the economically active age groups, the nation's expenditure on fish importation is too high enough to put tangible developmental projects to the nation. This is despite the natural resources which favour fisheries production from both aquaculture and wild capture sources. For the purpose of this chapter, the authors are interested in the domestic fish sources which come from aquaculture, artisanal fishing and industrial fishing. All these sources are with their unique work-related hazards which affect the health and general wellbeing of those who take part in them. As hazards can occur during the different stages of the fisheries value chain (production, processing, handling, storage and transportation), occupational hazards is treated in this chapter in totality as it affects all the value chain actors in the Nigerian fisheries sector.

The remaining of this chapter is structured under the preceding headings: overview of occupational hazards, classification of occupational hazards, fisheries in Nigeria, occupational hazards in fisheries, and empirical evidence of occupational hazards in fisheries in Nigeria.

2. Methods

Information used in this chapter was obtained through the desk review of published journals, conference proceedings and books as well as personal experiences of the authors with fish farmers, fishers and fish processors over time. The published materials were mainly sourced from the internet. While review studies from year 2000 were considered, only recent materials from Nigeria between 2011 and 2020 utilized in providing empirical evidences of occupational hazards in fisheries.

3. Linking occupational health to sustainable development

In this section, the authors first reviewed different literatures on the definition of health, occupation and occupational health. Occupational hazard was also defined as a concept and different categories were later identified and presented.

3.1 Definition of occupational health

Health is defined as a condition of complete physical, mental and social well-being which does not mean the mere absence of disease and infirmity. Health is associated to the physical conditions of both mind and body, of all people at the workplace including the workers, contractors and visitors, and their protection from harm in the form of injury or disease [11]. Occupational health is a branch of medicine concerned with the prevention and treatment/control of job-related injuries and illnesses. It is closely linked to public health and health systems development. According to WHO [12], occupational health is a multidisciplinary field of healthcare which deals with all aspects of health and safety, in order to enable a worker to discharge their occupational responsibilities, in a way that causes least harm to their health. This is achieved through the prevention of hazards.

According to the definition jointly provided by International Labour Organization and World Health Organization [13], the aims of occupational health include promoting and maintaining the highest level of physical, mental and social well-being of workers in all occupations; preventing amongst workers of departures from health caused by their working conditions; protecting the workers in their employment from risks resulting from factors adverse to health; the placing and maintenance of the worker in an occupational environment adapted to his physiological and psychological capabilities; and, above all, the adaptation of work to man and of each man to his job.

3.2 Health, work and sustainable development

Health is central to the sustainable development of nations globally, hence ensuring healthy living and promoting wellbeing of people has been included as a whole goal in the sustainable development agenda [14]. According to Alamu [15], sustainable development is the organizing principle for meeting human development goals while at the same time sustaining the ability of natural systems to provide the natural resources and ecosystems services upon which the economy and society depends. WHO [16] defined sustainable development as a strategy for meeting the present generation's needs without compromising the future generation's ability of meeting their needs. This implies that globally, human health is recognized as a prerequisite for the attainment of sustainable and productive economy.

In terms of occupational health, the attainment of sustainable development implies the satisfaction of material needs through work and other production processes without causing danger to one's health, environment, as well as the community resource base in both short and long terms. Occupational health is a basic element and constitutes a social and health dimension of the principle of sustainable development.

It could be summarized that unsafe and unhealthy workplace environment, especially in terms of poor ventilation, inappropriate lighting, excessive noise among others, affect workers performance [17].

4. Overview of occupational hazards

Before proceeding, it is important to define and/or explain some key terms such as occupation, and hazard. According to Dictionary.com, occupation refers to any activity or vocation in which a person is engaged. It also means a person's usual work or business which serves as a means of earning a living. Hazards refer to anything that has the potential of causing harm to people, environment and/or properties. A hazard is an unpleasant or undesirable event, situation or condition that takes place and has adverse effects on people. That is, any event that poses some level of potential threat or risk to life, health, property and the environment. While hazard is something that can cause harm, a risk is the chance that a hazard could harm somebody. To Ahmed, Dosoki and Nasr [18], hazard refers to the presence of materials or conditions that have the tendency to cause loss or harm or a combination of the severity of consequences and likelihood of occurrence of undesired outcomes. Based on this background, Breeding [19] defined occupational hazards as risks, illnesses or accidents that take place in the workplace. That is, unpleasant situations experienced by workers while doing their job. While making their contribution on the subject, Ford and Tetrick [20] described occupational hazard as an aspect of one's occupation-specific context that increases one's risk of injury. Any working condition that can lead to illness or death is an occupational hazard [21].

Hazards can occur at any time and at any place depending on the complexities of the work situation, environment and equipment used. Occupational hazards could result from the nature of materials/equipment being used, environment under which work is being done as well as the people involved in specific activities. Sadullah and Kanten [22] also classified the causes of occupational hazards into unsafe work conditions and unsafe behaviors. The fisheries industry like other agricultural activities especially in the developing countries is one that involves people of different age categories such as children and adults. Hazards are likely to occur more with children as they are not physically and psychologically matured enough to take part in fisheries operations. The use of inappropriate equipment by workers in the fisheries industry could even make adults vulnerable to occupational hazards. In fisheries, hazards could occur during harvesting/fish capture, processing, and handling and even during transportation of fish.

In relation to occupational health and safety, primary categories of hazards have been identified by authors as physical, chemical, biological, ergonomic and behavioural hazards [23–24].

4.1 Physical hazards

Physical hazards are materials, substances or activities that threaten a worker's physical safety. According to Harwood [25], physical hazards involve environmental hazards that can cause harm with or without contact. They are injuries that occur on one's body parts such as hands, eyes, legs, etc. They are often the most common in any workplace. They include noise, heat and cold stress, bruises from fall, illumination, vibration, and electromagnetic radiation.

Some of the physical hazards are pictorially shown in **Figures 1–5** below.

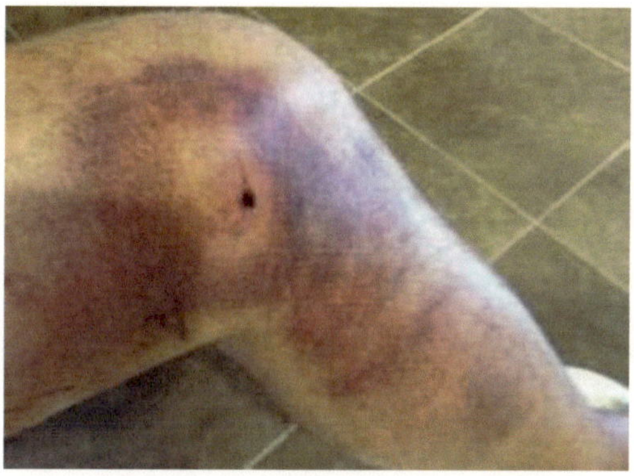

Figure 1.
Bruise from fall. ***Source:*** *www.ibtimes.com cited in Olaoye et al. [26].*

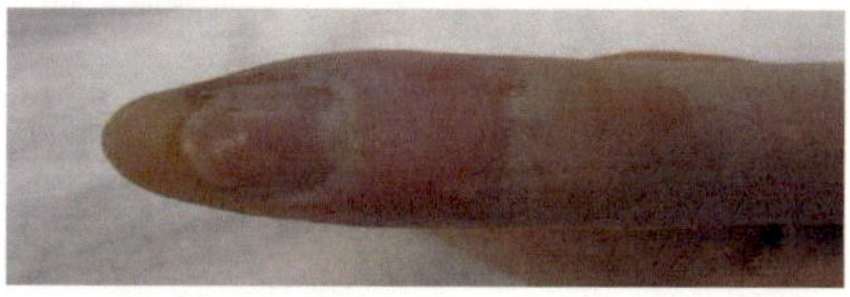

Figure 2.
Whitlow (finger infection). ***Source:*** *www.emedicinehealth.com/fingerinfection/articleem.htm cited in Olaoye et al. [26].*

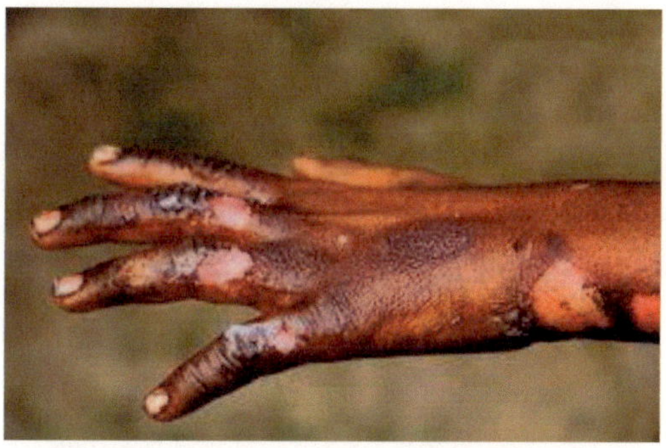

Figure 3.
Burn injuries. ***Source:*** *www.elginburninjurylawyer.co cited in Olaoye et al. [26].*

4.2 Chemical hazards

These are subtype of occupational hazards resulting from exposure to harmful and dangerous chemical compounds. Chemicals in the form of solids, liquids, gases, fumes, dusts, mists and vapour could have toxic effects on workers if inhaled through breathing, direct contact with the skin (absorption), or ingested by eating or drinking [5]. Hazardous chemicals include neurotoxins, immune agents, dermatologic toxins, systemic toxins, pneumoconiotic agents, and sensitizers.

4.3 Biological hazards

These are hazards in the workplace caused by biological agents such as microorganisms and toxins produced by living organisms [26]. They exist in exposure to bacteria, virus, fungi and other living organisms. Fisheries and other occupations

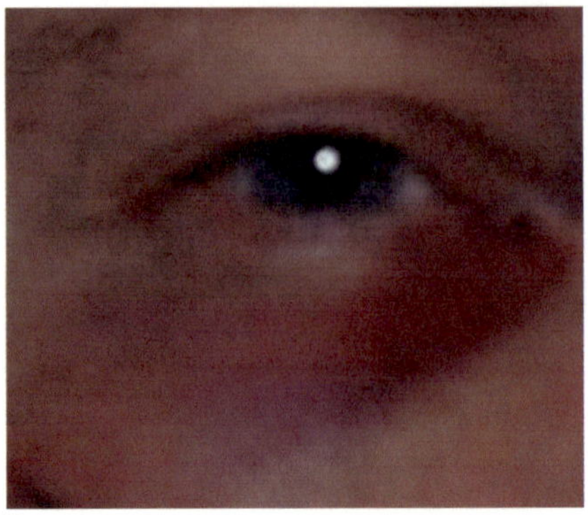

Figure 4.
Red eye injury. ***Source:*** *www.letsgohealthy.blogspot.com cited in Olaoye et al. [26].*

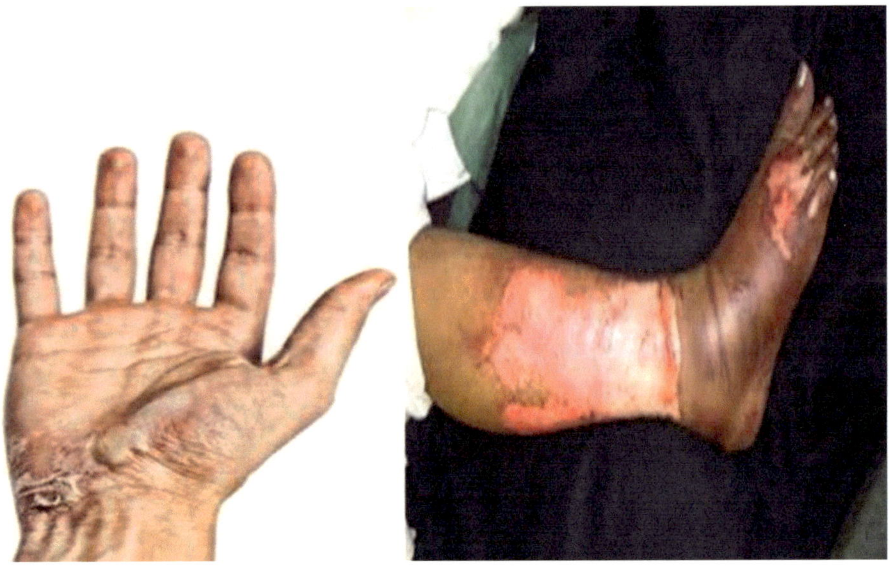

Figure 5.
Hand and leg burn. ***Source:*** *www.besthealthybodycare.com cited in Olaoye et al. [26].*

that expose workers to plants and animals or their products are prone to biological hazards. Examples of biological hazards include bites and stings from snakes, insects, scorpions and spiders.

4.4 Psychosocial/behaviour hazards

As the name implies, psychosocial hazards are a subtype of occupational hazards which affects a person's social life or psychological health. These include occupational burnout, and occupational stress. It could be manifested from boredom, production pressure, repetitive tasks, and low pay.

4.5 Ergonomic hazard

The science of fitting jobs to workers instead of trying to get the worker to fit the job is known as ergonomics. The occupational hazards resulting from the workstation design and tools are ergonomic hazards. These include fatigue and injury, extreme temperature, discomfort, and pain. It could ultimately lead to musculoskeletal disorder.

5. Fisheries in Nigeria

Fisheries refers to the science of producing fish and other aquatic resources for the purpose of providing food for humans and livestock, recreational fishing, and obtaining ornamental fish or fish products such as fish oil [27]. This definition refers to the production of fish and other living organisms in water bodies for the benefit of mankind through consumption, commercial or recreational purposes. In Nigeria, fisheries as a concept is divided into capture and culture fisheries with the capture fisheries further divided into artisanal and industrial fisheries. Artisanal fishery is to the harvesting or capturing of fishes from natural water bodies and ponds by small scale fisher folks using primarily the traditional fishing gears [28]. Some authors [29, 30] regarded it as a nonindustrial fishery covering the activities of small-scale canoes operating in the coastal areas, creeks, lagoons, inshore water, and the inland rivers. The artisanal fishery, though involves the use of crude implements, with little or no access to credit, and subsistence level of operation, contributes the bulkiest proportion up to 90 percent of domestic fish production in Nigeria [31–33].

The industrial fisheries are a higher and mechanized level of fish production, which relies heavily on the use of trawling vessels for fishing and shrimping in the territorial and offshore waters [34]. By this definition, it could be implied that industrial fishery is highly capital intensive and involves the use of advanced technologies. As such, it could only be practiced by insignificantly few people. No wonder, Moses [35] submitted that artisanal fishery employs 18 times more fishermen than the industrial fishery. Aquaculture has been defined as the rearing of aquatic organisms (e.g. fish, insects, bivalves, mollusks, crustaceans, and aquatic plants) under controlled or semi-controlled environments (such as ponds, pens, raceways and cages) for the social and economic benefits of mankind and livestock [36, 37].

In Nigeria, although domestic fish production is on the increase, the ever-increasing population of the country makes the country a net importer of fish and fish products despite the contribution of both the aquaculture and artisanal fisheries components. Despite the fact that artisanal fishery contributes more to local fish production, one could summarize from different Nigerian fisheries statistics that while production from the capture fisheries is relatively on the decline, production from aquaculture remains on the increase. This was supported by FAO [38] that aquaculture production has been on the increase since 1995. This is why Olaoye et al. [39] regarded aquaculture as the fastest growing livestock production sector in Nigeria. Supporting this claim, Giwa et al. [40] while investigating the trends of fish production in Nigeria submitted that artisanal fishery contributed 77.95 percent of the domestic fish production and that aquaculture maintains the highest growth rate of 12.53 percent.

The fisheries sub-sector has been recognized as a major economic component, with an estimate of employing more than 8.6 million people directly and additional 19.6 million indirectly [41].

6. Occupational hazards in fisheries: Empirical evidences from Nigeria

Although occupational health, hazards and safety are the concern of many government agencies and international organizations such as the World Health Organization – WHO, Food and Agriculture Organization - FAO and the International Labour Organization- ILO especially with respect to working in the agriculture sector, little empirical evidences abound on the prevalence of occupational hazards in Nigeria. Where available, data are mostly not disaggregated by subsectors. More importantly, there is dearth of information on occupational hazards associated with the fisheries industry. Apart from the general hazards associated with the agriculture sector, workers in the fishery subsector are exposed to other numerous hazards related to water impoundments, transportation, shift and night-time work and offshore operations [42].

6.1 Occupational hazards in aquaculture

According to Erondu and Anyanwu [24], hazards in aquaculture can be classified into physical, chemical and biological. Physical risk factors in the aquaculture industry include injuries such as stings from fish spines, cuts, sprains, fractures, asthma and rhinitis, snake bites, crab crawling and bites from fish as well as mechanical injuries associated with laboratories. Physical hazards in the aquaculture industry could mainly be in form of noise, injuries and asthma [24].

The use of locally fabricated equipment/machines in most of the feedmills in Nigeria exposes the workers to excessive noise which results in loss of hearing and mental fatigue. Some fish species such as *Clarias gariepinus, Protopterus aethiopicus, Barbus intermedius, Oreochromis niloticus, Baringoensis* and *Lado cylindricus* have fins which can prick fish farmers and their workers if not handled with care [26]. According to Dorooshi [43], Catfish species have strong pectoral fins with spines which are capable of pricking fish farmers as well as sharp teeth used in biting workers during sorting and harvesting in the aquaculture industry. The biting and pricking caused by fish spines and sharp teeth could lead to injuries which are mainly non-fatal but according to Olaoye [26], can lead to amputation of fingers if exposed to viral and bacterial infections. Cuts resulting from the use of sharp objects such as knives and oyster shell are additional causes of injuries [24]. Erondu and Anyanwu [24] also noted that needle stick injury could result among hatchery workers. Aquaculture workers in the feedmill are also prone to asthma caused by dusts from the mixture of different food particles including flour. According to Karkkainen [44], dust released from flour and animal feedmill is the second most common cause of asthma.

Aquaculture workers are also exposed to chemical hazards as a result of inorganic fertilizers, lime, pesticides and formaldehyde in fish ponds; acute and chronic pollution of water ways; flocculants, and disinfectants. The biological hazards in aquaculture include parasitic infestation and pathogenic infections.

6.2 Occupational hazards in artisanal fishing

Like the aquaculture component, the artisanal fishery is also inherently associated with numerous hazards. In fact, fishing seems to be riskier than aquaculture. According to Oyediran *et al.* [45], fishers are vulnerable due to depleting stock arising from over fishing and excessive pressures on available resources, environmental degradation due to flooding, deforestation and menace of water hyacinth. Industrial activities such as oil spillage, canalization, construction of hydroelectric dams also destabilize ecosystems and fishing activities thereby posing serious occupational hazards to fishers.

Just like with the workers in the aquaculture industry, fisherfolks in the artisanal fishery sector are exposed to injuries caused by bites and pricks from sharp fish spines and fins [9, 45]. Additionally, most if not all the fishermen in Nigeria still makes use of hook and line or longline. The fisherfolks can also sustain injuries when trying to remove the hooks from harvested fish and when attaching baits onto the hooks [46]. The tasks of the workers in artisanal fishery include repetitive lifting and pulling of heavy fish loads into fishing vessels, and offloading [8, 47]. These result into musculoskeletal injuries [10].

Fisherfolks mostly work under harsh conditions of either extreme hot or cold weather. Working under hot weather conditions exposes the fisherfolks to sun radiation from the sun thereby causing skin burn. According to Kennedy et al. [48] and Coups *et al.* [49], exposure to sun rays causes skin cancer. Working under extremely cold condition on rainy days could result into respiratory problems such as sneezing and coughing.

Since artisanal fishery is attributed with the use of obnoxious fishing methods such as the use of chemicals and explosives, water bodies are both polluted and destroyed thereby affecting artisanal fishing. According to their findings, Oyediran *et al.* [50] identified flood disasters, physical injuries, stings and bites, cuts and wounds, and leach attack as the most common occupational health hazards in artisanal fish production. According to them, considerable income and man-days are lost as a result of occupational health hazards. Udolisa *et al.* [9] also researched into the occupational and health hazards in Nigerian coastal fisheries while using the mixed method of data collection. The authors summarized that coastal artisanal fisheries in Nigeria is associated with body injuries such as cuts, fish bites, fire injuries, and foundering.

6.3 Occupational hazards in fish processing

Fish processing is a phase/stage in the fish value chain associated with fish and fish products between the time of harvest and the time of delivering the final product to the consumer [51]. Fish processing includes smoking, chilling and freezing, canning, and the production of other value-added products [23–24, 52–53]. Apart from minimizing postharvest losses of fish, fish processing adds to the nutritive value of the fish [54].

Various hazards have been reported in fish processing industry which ranges from redness/swelling of the eye (which is the commonest) to mechanical and electrical accidents, bacterial and parasitic infections, noise induced hearing loss, allergic respiratory diseases and stress related health problems. Processors and other workers in the fish processing industry are susceptible to many hazards while doing their work [26]. Following the review of previous literatures [23], occupational hazards in fish processing are discussed under physical, chemical, biological, ergonomic, and psychosocial hazards.

Physical hazards in fish processing include minor cuts and scrapes resulting from the use of knives and other sharp tools, falls caused by slippery floors, burns, hypertension, eye disease, stings from fish spines arising when one is handling fish without the use of appropriate safety devices, whitlow resulting from bacterial or fungal infection of the tip of one's finger and/or toe, exposure to heat and cold leading to headache, sneezing and/or coughing, eye injury such as redness of the eye, burns, head injury, and bruising [54]. Redness of the eye results when the eye have direct contact with the smoke especially during smoking or frying fish with local/traditional kilns that make use of fuel woods thereby leading to the eye surface being red [23]. It is associated with itching, mucus discharge, pain or even blurred vision.

According to Norwegian Labor Inspection Authority [55], sprain and fracture could be caused by slippery floors and stairs when carrying loads and materials while processing fish. Although Udolisa *et al.* [9] noted that injuries from minor cuts and scrapes due to their non-fatal nature does not lead to prolonged loss of work, it is important to treat cuts and wounds so as not to expose them to infections. Stings from fish can sometimes be poisonous and cause severe pains especially when exposed to tetanus infection [23].

Handling of fish in preparation for processing involves the dipping of hands in cold water even on rainy days for a long time resulting in respiratory irritation such as sneezing and coughing, blanching and sores in the hands which could lead to whitlow on the tips of the fingers and at times, toes [23]. According to authors [26, 56–57], whitlow is a serious fungal or bacterial infection which is very painful and can result to amputation of the finger, toe or nail. Headache, fatigue and general weakness of the body could also be the consequences under the sun, in extreme heat or with cold water for too long.

In Nigeria, fish processing is characterized with low level of mechanization which involves the use of fuel woods for smoking and/or frying of fish [51, 58]. The implication includes that the fish processors and their workers spend reasonably long duration (mostly from morning till night) in the open under the radiation from sunlight. Since smoking is the commonest method of processing fish in Nigeria [39, 51], the fish processors are highly exposed to smoke fire/naked flame of extremely high temperature which has adverse effect on the health of the fish processors [59]. The report of Adei *et al.* [59] submitted that work-related injuries and diseases resulted in the loss of 7% of the total annual income of the fish processors in 2016.Noise and/or vibration is another important physical hazards associated with fish processing as fish processors are frequently exposed to noise and vibrations at landing sites. This has the tendency to cause either temporary or permanent hearing impairment depending on the level of exposure [9].

Biological hazards that fish processors are exposed to especially while harvesting fish from ponds without wearing protective clothing include parasites (leeches, nematodes, cestodes) and pathogenic infections such as *Vibrio vulnificus* [59]. According to Kolndadacha *et al.* [60], infectious diseases caused by virus, fungi, bacteria and even protozoa can be transmitted by farmers as a result of handling fish or eating improperly cooked fish.

The chemical hazards associated with fish processing include principally the inhalation of smoke which can cause asthma and other respiratory ailments. Fish processors could also be exposed to smoke particles that contain potential or confirmed carcinogens such as polycyclic aromatic hydrocarbons – PAHs [61]. The use of disinfectants such as formalin and Gamalin 20 also poses health hazards to consumers of fish because of residual effect [23]. Ergonomic hazards associated with fish processing include internal injuries of the liver, spleen, stomach, colon, pancreas and blood vessels which can be caused by motor vehicle accidents, blunt trauma or penetrating injuries [62]. Broken bone/dislocation, back strain and sprain are additional ergonomic hazards faced by fish processors.

In fish processing, psychosocial hazards result from prolonged work and mental demand. According to the review made by Mshelia *et al.* [23], extra hours of work might put fish processors at a greater risk of depression. Handling an insane amount of workload lately is definitely an act of inching towards depression which gives room for the occurrence of other hazards. Studies have suggested the symptoms of prolonged work to include appetite loss, disturbed sleep, constantly sulking, muscle fatigue, loss of energy, indecisiveness, and poor concentration at work [63]. The mental demand is the potent force in achievement as the attitude of the mind affects the expression of the face, determines action, changes our physical condition and regulates our lives [64].

An empirical evidence of hazards associated with fish processing was provided through a study by Olaoye *et al.* [54], whose findings revealed that the working condition of artisanal fish processors was generally poor as majority of the fish processors reported that they worked frequently with poorly designed equipment, poorly maintained facilities, poorly constructed equipment, under constrained neck posture, and with poor hand tools. The most common category of the hazards

Occupational hazards	Artisanal fishing	Aquaculture	Fish processing
Noise/vibration	Common	Common	Common
Stings/bites from fish	Common	Common	Common
Cuts from knives and other sharp objects	Not common	Common	Common
Wounds from fishing gears (longlines, hook and line)	Common	Not common	Not common
Asthma	Not common	Common	Common
Musculoskeletal injuries	Common	Common	Common
Skin cancer	Common	Not common	Common
Redness of eye	Not common	Not common	Common
Respiratory problems (sneezing, coughing)	Common	Common	Common
Skin burns	Not common	Not common	Common
Chemical hazards	Common	Common	Common
Biological hazards	Common	Common	Not common
Psychosocial hazards	Common	Common	Common

Table 1.
Summary of occupational hazards in artisanal fishing, aquaculture and fish processing.

associated with fish smoking, according to Olaoye *et al.* [54] is the chemical hazards (exposure to smoke, fumes and gases). From one of the studies of Dhakal and Nayak [65], musculoskeletal symptoms were reportedly experienced by majority of the fish processors, and that musculoskeletal problems were promoted by faulty body posture, repetitive activity, and poor condition of the work environment.

To Ibrahim *et al.* [66], the major occupational hazards among fish processors in Nassarawa State, Nigeria were redness and/or swelling of the eye. In supporting this report, Olopade [67] reported skin rashes and redness of the eye as the major occupational hazards among small scale women fish processors around Asejire Dam of Oyo State, Nigeria.

Occupational hazards common in artisanal fisheries, aquaculture and fish processing were compared in terms of prevalence as summarized in **Table 1**.

7. Conclusions

Review of literature on occupational hazards associated with fisheries has shown that fisheries like other components of agriculture is a very risky venture which can lead to severe injuries and eventual death if workers' health is not protected and promoted within the industry. It further indicated that although the different value chains are affected by different hazards at varying levels depending on level of exposure and scale of operation as well as the adherence to safety in the workplace, the fisheries industry is vulnerable to physical, chemical, biological, ergonomic and psychosocial hazards. Occupational hazards generally have negative effects on the level of production of fish, revenue from fisheries, and loss of man-days. The authors recommend that:

1. Awareness should be raised among workers and employees in the fisheries industry on occupational safety and health. The awareness should focus on the associated risks and hazards;

2. Stakeholders (fish farmers, fishermen, fish processors, etc) should be encouraged to make available and use personal protective gears while working. Employers in the industry should be compelled to make protective gears available to their employees, and enforce the use of such gears in order to reduce accidents;

3. First aid kits should be a prerequisite in all landing sites, aquaculture facilities, and processing plants. The workers should also be educated on the proper use of the first aid kits in case of accidents in the course of working.

4. Obnoxious fishing methods should be discouraged by strictly sanctioning defaulters;

5. Researchers should delve into studies on occupational health hazards in aquaculture, artisanal fishing, industrial fishing, fish processing, and even fish marketing. These researches, if well conducted, reported and disseminated, will provide an update on the different categories of health hazards in fisheries especially with Nigeria in focus.

Conflicts of interest

The authors hereby declare that there is no conflict of interest in this chapter preparation.

Author details

Olalekan Jacob Olaoye[1] and Wahab Gbenga Ojebiyi[2*]

1 Agricultural Media Resources and Extension Center, Federal University of Agriculture, Abeokuta, Nigeria

2 Department of Agricultural Extension and Rural Development, Federal University of Agriculture, Abeokuta, Nigeria

*Address all correspondence to: oluwagbemiga2013@gmail.com

References

[1] Park K. Park's Textbook of Preventive and Social Medicine, 21st Edition. M/s Banarsidas Bhanot Publishers. 2011.1167, Prem Nagar, Jabalpur, 482 001 (M.P.) India.

[2] Olowogbon ST. Health and Safety in Agriculture and Food Security Nexus. International Journal of Emerging Sciences, 2011; **1**(2): 73-82.

[3] Adedeji IA, Olapade-Ogunwole F, Farayola CO, Adejumo IO. Productivity effects of occupational hazards among poultry farmers and farm workers in Osogbo Local Government Area of Osun State. International Journal of Poultry Science. 2011; **10**(11): 867-870.

[4] Idio AD, Adejare GT. Conceptual analysis of rural farmers' health and its implication on agricultural productivity. Nigerian Journal of Agriculture, Food and Environment. 2013; **8**(3):32-38.

[5] World Health Organization - WHO. Occupational health: A manual for primary health care workers. World Health Organization Regional Office for the Eastern Mediterranean. 2001; 44p.

[6] Egbetokun OA, Ajijola S, Omonona BT, Omidele MA. Farmers' health and technical efficiency in Osun State Nigeria. International Journal of Food and Nutrition Science. 2012; **1**(1): 13-30.

[7] Hawkes C, Ruel MT. The links between agriculture and health: an inter-sectorial opportunity to improve the health and livelihoods of the poor. Bulletin of the World Health Organization. 2006; **84**(12): 985-991.

[8] Frantzeskou E, Kastania AN, Riza E, Jensen OC, Linos A. Risk factors for fishermen's health and safety in Greece. International Maritime Health. 2012; **63**:155-161.

[9] Udolisa REK, Akinyemi AA, Olaoye OJ. Occupational and health hazards in Nigerian coastal artisanal fisheries. Journal of Fisheries and Aquatic Science. 2013; **8**:14-20.

[10] Global Burden Disease – GBD. Mortality and Causes of Death Collaborators. Global, regional, and national life expectancy, all-cause mortality, and cause specific mortality for 249 causes of death. 1980-2015: a systematic analysis for the Global Burden of Disease Study 2015. *Lancet*. 2015;388:1459-1544.

[11] Khan WA, Mustaq T, Tabassum A. Occupational health, safety and risk analysis. International Journal of Science, Environment and Technology. 2014; **3**(4): 1336-1346.

[12] World Health Organization – WHO. Global Strategy on Occupational Health for All Organisation. The Way to Health at Work. Geneva, Switzerland: WHO. 2015.

[13] International Labour Organization, World Health Organization. Occupational health services and practice. 1994; Ilo.org. Retrieved 2015-04-15.

[14] Akpama SI, Bessong CD, Bessong NO. Attainment of the sustainable development goals (SDGs): The relevance of adult basic education. Education for Today. 2017; **13**(1): 13-19.

[15] Alamu O. Sustainable development goals in Nigeria: What roles for Nigeria's indigenous languages? European Journal of Research and Reflection in Educational Sciences. 2017; **5**(4): 1-13.

[16] World Health Organization – WHO. Occupational health – Global strategies on occupational health for all: The way to health at work. Recommendation

of the second meeting of the WHO Collaborating Centres in Occupational Health, 11-14 October 1994, Beijing, China.

[17] Chandrasekar K. Workplace environment and its impact on organisational performance in public sector organisations. International Journal of Enterprise Computing and Business Systems. 2011; **1**(1) Retrieved December 20, 2014 from http://www.ijecbs.com/January2015.

[18] Ahmed ZAM, Dosoki MI, Nasr SAA. Occupational hazards in fish industry. World Journal of Fish and Marine Science. 2012; **4**(2): 201-210.

[19] Breeding DC. What is hazardous? Occupational Health and Safety. Retrieved from https://ohsonline.com>2011/07/01

[20] Ford MT, Tetrick LE. Relations among occupational hazards, attitudes and safety performance. Journal of Occupational Health Psychology. 2011; **16**(1): 48-66.

[21] International Labour Organization - ILO. International Labour Office: Safety and health in agriculture, Published by SafeWork, International Labour Office. 2000; 4, route de Morillons CH-1211 Geneva 22 – Switzerland. https://pdfs.semanticscholar.org/1c16/dd6ee54584f42c1cbceb5d8cdb471f6514e2.pdf. Accessed 01/02/2017

[22] Sadullah O, Kanten S. A research on the effect of organizational safety climate upon the safe behaviors. Ege Academic Review. 2009; **9**(3): 923-932.

[23] Mshelia MB, Bassey JU, Wanas NL, Garba U. A review of some potential occupational, environmental hazards and injuries associated with fish production in Nigeria. African Scholar Journal of Agriculture and Agricultural Technology. 2019; **15**(1): 72-88.

[24] Erondu ES, Anyanwu PE. Potential hazards and risks associated with the aquaculture industry. African Journal of Biotechnology. 2005; **4** (13): 1622-1627.

[25] Harwood S. Grant products by topic. 2015. Available at www.osha.gov.

[26] Olaoye OJ, Odebiyi OC, Abimbola OT. Occupational hazards and injuries associated with fish processing in Nigeria. Journal of Aquatic Science. 2015; **3**(1): 1-5. doi: 10.12691/jas-3-1-1.

[27] IGI Global. *What is fisheries?* 2020. Retrieved from www.igi-global.com on August 25, 2020.

[28] Okwu OJ, Yahaya MA, Obinne CPO. Analysis of artisanal fisher folk information needs and accessibility in Benue State, Nigeria. Asian Journal of Agricultural Sciences. 2011;**3**(5):408-413

[29] Baruwa OI, Tijani AA, Adejobi AO. Profitability and constraints to fishery enterprises: A case of artisanal and aquaculture fisheries in Lagos State, Nigeria. Nigerian Journal of Agriculture, Food and Environment. 2012;**8**(1):52-58

[30] Olatunji AE, Olah OM. The socio-economic status of artisanal fishers in Cross River, Cross River State, Nigeria. World Journal of Fish and Marine Sciences. 2012;**4**(6):672-678. DOI: 10.5829/idosi.wjfms.2012.04.06.668

[31] Olaoye OJ, Ojebiyi WG. Marine fisheries in Nigeria: A review. In: Marine ecology: Biotic and abiotic interactions. Intech Open. 2018; 155-173. http://dx.doi.org/10.5772/intechopen.75032.

[32] Adepegba OB. Improving fish processing and marketing in Nigeria. A paper presented at a National Stakeholders workshop on inland capture fisheries Development, the women development centre, Kaduna. Feb 20-22, 2007. 23 p

[33] Ajekigbe JM. Fisheries development in Nigeria: The challenges and prospects of accessing funds. Being lecture presented at the annual public lecture of the Fisheries Society of Nigeria, organized by FISON at Nigerian Institute for International affairs, Victoria Island Lagos Jul 12, 2007. 23 p

[34] Dada BF. Contribution of fisheries to employment national economy and food security in Nigeria. A paper presented by Honourable Minister of State for Agricultural and Rural Development presented at the 2003 FISON Lecture, Lagos Dec 22, 2003. Fish Network a Quarterly Publication of FISON; 2003. 21 p

[35] Moses BS. Tropical Fisheries. Kaduna: Abaam Publishing Co., 2002. 26 p

[36] Tunde AB, Kuton MP, Oladipo AA, Olasunkanmi LH. Economic analyze of costs and return of fish farming in Saki-east local government area of Oyo State, Nigeria. Journal of Aquaculture Resources Development. 2015;**6**(2):306-310

[37] Nandi AS, Gunn P, Adegboye GA, Barnabas TM. Assessment of fish farmers' livelihood and poverty status in Delta State, Nigeria. Agriculture, Forestry and Fisheries. 2014; **3**(5):427-433.

[38] Food and Agriculture Organization – FAO. The State of World Fisheries and Aquaculture 2016. Contributing to Food Security and Nutrition for All. Rome. 2016. 200p

[39] Olaoye OJ, Ojebiyi WG, Opele AI, Baiyewu AK. Socioeconomic analysis of small scale fish farmers in Ilaro agricultural extension zone of Ogun State, Nigeria. Journal of Agriculture, Forestry and Fisheries. 2016;**15**(2):64-74

[40] Giwa EJ, Jim-Saiki L, Adeyemo AM, Unah RL, Waniko SN, Ogunbadejo HK, Alhaji T. Short-term prediction of fish production in Nigeria: Empirical study Nigeria fish demand and supply. International Journal of Advanced Multidisciplinary Research. 2018; **5**(9): 28-37.

[41] WorldFish. WorldFish Nigeria Strategy: 2018-2022. Penang, Malaysia: WorldFish. 2018; Strategy: 2018-09.

[42] Myers ML. Review of occupational hazards associated with aquaculture. Journal of Agromedicine. 2010;15:412-426.

[43] Dorooshi G. Catfish stings: a report of two cases. Journal of Research in Medical Sciences. 2012; **17**: 578-581.

[44] Karkkainen E. When work becomes a wheeze. World health safety. . 2002; 12p.

[45] Oijen MJP. Appendix I. Key to Lake Victoria fishes other than haplochromine cichlids. In: Witte F and van Densen WLT, eds. *Fish Stocks and Fisheries of Lake Victoria. A Handbook for Field Observations*. Dyfed, UK: Samara Publishing Limited; 1995:209-300

[46] Ngaruiya FW, Oghendi GM, Mokua MA. Occupational health risks and hazards among the fisherfolk in Kampi Samaki, Lake Baringo, Kenya. Environmental Health Insights. 2019; **13**: 1-11.

[47] Novalbos J, Nogueroles P, Soriguer M, Piniella F. Occupational health in the Andalusian fisheries sector. Occupational Medicine (Lond). 2008; **58**:141-143.

[48] Kennedy C, Bajdik CD, Willemze R, De Gruijl FR, Bouwes Bavinck JN. The influence of painful sunburns and lifetime sun exposure on the risk of actinic keratoses, seborrheic warts, melanocytic nevi, atypical nevi, and

skin cancer. Journal of Investigative Dermatology. 2003; **120**:1087-1093.

[49] Coups EJ, Manne SL, Heckman CJ. Multiple skin cancer risk behaviors in the US population. American Journal of Preventive Medicine. 2008; **34**:87-93.

[50] Oyediran W, Sodiya C, Omoare A, Ogbonna C. Effects of Occupational Health Hazards on Artisanal Fish Production in Ogun State, Nigeria. Fish and Ocean Opj. 2017; **3**(2): 001-006.

[51] Adeyeye SAO. Traditional fish processing in Nigeria: a critical review. Nutrition and Food Science. 2016; **46**(3): 321-336.

[52] Myers ML. Aquaculture safety and health: Review. University of Kentucky College of Public Health. Southeast Center for Agricultural Health and Injury Prevention. 2008.

[53] Ezekiel EN, Abowei JFN, Ezekiel EF. Hazard and risk analysis in culture fisheries. Research Journal of Applied Sciences, Engineering and Technology. 2011; **3**(10): 1108-1117.

[54] Olaoye OJ, Ojebiyi WG, Ogunremi JB, Oose MO, Ojeikhoa OR, Opele AI. Some hazardous practices associated with artisanal fish processing in Ogun Waterside Local Government Area of Ogun State, Nigeria. Applied Tropical Agriculture. 2017; **22**(1): 68-77.

[55] Norwegian Labor Inspection Authority. Work environment and safety in aquaculture: Tips for risk assessment and precautionary measures. A booklet (Translated from Norwegian). Trondheim, Norway: Norwegian Labor Inspection Authority. 2001.

[56] Anh VT, Van der Hock W, Ersboll AK, Vicheth C, Cam PD, Dalsgaard A, Peri-urbam. Aquatic plant culture and skin disease in Phnom Penh Cambodia. Journal of Water Health. 2009; 7:302-311.

[57] Trang do T, Moibak K, Cam PD, Dalsgard A. Incidence of and risk factor for skin ailment among farmers working with waste water-fed agriculture in Hawaii, Vietnam. Transactions of the Royal Society of Tropical Medicine and Hygien. 2007; **101**:502-510.

[58] Davies RM, Davies OA. Traditional and improved fish processing technologies in Bayelsa State, Nigeria. European Journal of Science Research. 2009; **26**: 539-548.

[59] Adei D, Braimah I, Mensah JV. Occupational health and safety practices among fish processors in Kumasi Metropolitan Area, Ghana. Occupational Health Science. 2019; **3**: 83-102.

[60] Kolndadacha OD, Musa YM, Okaeme AN, Ibiwoye TII, Nyaku RE. Occupational and environmental hazards associated with fish production. 2015.

[61] Cole DW, Cole R, Gaydos SJ, Gray J, Hyland G, Jacques ML, Powell-Dunford N, Sawhney C, Au WW. Aquaculture:environmental,toxicological and health issues. International Journal of Hygiene and Environmental Health. 2009; **212**: 369-377.

[62] Claussen CB. High accident rates in aquaculture. Gemini. 2011; Accessed on 07.26.2000 at http://www.ntnu.no/gemini/2000-06e/10.htm.

[63] Moreau DTR, Neis B. Occupational health and safety hazards in Atlantic Canadian aquaculture: Laying the groundwork for prevention. Marine Policy. 2009; **33**: 401-411.

[64] Myers ML. Addressing risks and benefits: emerging technologies assessed for safety and health of farming people. Resource. 2005; **12**: 13-14.

[65] Dhakal H, Nayak MG. Occupational health problems and factors contributing to the problem among fisherwomen. International Journal of Advanced Research in Biological Sciences. 2015; **2**(5): 169-176.

[66] Ibrahim HI, Kigbu AA, Mohammed R. Women's experiences in small scale fish processing in Lake Feferuwa fishing community, Nassarawa State, Nigeria. Livestock research for Rural Development. 2011; **23**(3): 11-18.

[67] Olopade OA. The socio-economic of small scale women fish processors around Asejire Dam of Oyo State. Spanish Journal of Rural Development. 2012; **3**(2): 59-65.

Chapter 3

Occupational Health and Safety Standards of Foreign Seasonal Farm Workers: Evaluation of Personal Protection Measures, Policies and Practices

Swarna Weerasinghe

Abstract

Health and safety standards are paramount to all agricultural workers and more so to the foreign seasonal farm workers. European, North American and Oceanic agricultural sector heavily depends on the foreign workers migrating temporarily to carryout seasonal agricultural work that are not attractive to local citizens. The aim of this chapter is to critically analyze existing workplace health and safety measures, policies and practices of Foreign agricultural workers with a secondary focus on Canadian public health standards that applies to COVID-19 pandemic control and beyond. During the pandemic, many countries opened international labour migration as a measure of economic recovery. Recent news media reported two Caribbean workers in the Canadian Agricultural sector, had died of COVID-19 complications. The basis of this chapter is the research based evidence that the author carried out on occupational health and safety standards of the population of foreign seasonal farm workers using a multi-method data collection: a scoping review of existing standards, policies and practices and personal interviews with seasonal agricultural workers and their employers. This chapter provides a critical analysis of data from multiple sources and from multiple jurisdictions to uncover gaps and malpractices of existing occupational health and safety practice standards for illness and injury prevention of foreign seasonal farm workers.

Keywords: foreign seasonal farm workers, farmers, workers' and NGO perspectives, agriculture work related health and safety, public health measures of COVID-19, illness and injury prevention

1. Introduction

There is a decade long worldwide trend of labour migration from the developing and underdeveloped countries to the developed countries. European, North American, and Oceanic agricultural sectors heavily depend on the foreign workers, migrating temporarily to carryout seasonal agricultural work that are not attractive to local citizens. Long work hours, low pay, hard work and hazardous work environments makes the agricultural sector unattractive to local labour force. Seasonal agricultural workers migrate to North America and Europe from developing and underdeveloped countries in the regions of South America, Caribbean, Africa, Eastern Europe and Asia with little or no prior training to gain knowledge about occupational health and safety guidelines and issues in the host country. Most of the seasonal agricultural workers to Canada and United States are from 11 Caribbean countries and Mexico [1]. There is abundance of research-based evidence merging from Europe, North America and Oceania confirming agricultural workers, in general, and foreign seasonal farm workers more specifically, as experiencing high occupational health associated health risks and injuries [2]. Focus of this chapter is to elucidate existing occupational health and safety standards and how these standards are applied to foreign seasonal farm workers, using case studies and interview data collected from Canada that offers a universal healthcare coverage to all permanent residents and citizens.

The term "foreign seasonal farm worker" refers to those temporary workers, who come under "work visa" to work in the farms, vegetation, animal husbandry, meat, or fish production facilities [1]. These foreign seasonal farm workers (FSFW) often get attracted to concentrations of agricultural facilities, where workers are paid minimal wages, work has to be carried out under hazardous conditions and workers are required to work long hours [2]. Due to those conditions and the work is only available seasonally, those jobs are unattractive to local people and often requires foreign workers to fill the essential labour shortage. It was reported in the year 2004 that of the 1.2 million farm workers in the United States, 12% of them were migrant workers [2]. In Finland 42% of the berry and vegetable picking industry relies on foreign seasonal farm workers [3]. Canadian agricultural sector heavily depends on the seasonal migrant workers and around 70,000 agricultural workforces (75% of the total agricultural labour force) during the period 2015–2017 were foreign seasonal farm workers [4].

Occupational health and workers' safety are inseparable issues, especially with regards to FSFWs since their occupational health issues of interest in this chapter are intrinsically related to lack of safety measures. FSFWs go through pre-migration medical screening prior to obtaining work VISA to enter into the host country. Those screening would prevent, those who have communicable diseases that threaten Canadian public and those who have disabilities, to migrate as temporary workers. Recent global pandemic has added a new dimension of public health related safety issues to the population of migrant workers. A section of this chapter will provide an overview of recent experience using a scoping review of gray literature and government reports. Through an occupational health and safety lens, this chapter illustrates a wide spectrum of issues; starting from the contractual agreements that impede equitable access to health and safety measures, through micro level migration related cultural and language issues to macro level housing and safety matters.

There is under reporting of injury and illnesses of FSFW due to the temporary nature of the work, language and cultural barriers [5] and these individuals' participation in the healthcare is minimal [6]. Underreporting of injuries and illnesses by the FSWF is partly due to fear of being deported or losing their job [5], in line with systemic structural issues. Two lists are maintained by employers who request foreign seasonal workers; a named list in which they specify the names of the workers whom they want to come back next year and then unnamed list where the liaison office from the sending country provide a list. In order to be in the named list, workers need to be the chosen ones from the previous employer and those who demand health and safety measures are unlikely to be chosen ones.

Two-year chart review in the United States reported 516 cases of work related injuries, over two seasons, that includes; muscle and joint strains (31%), falling (18%), object strikes (8%), and poison IV contacts (10%) [6]. There are considerable number of female FSFWs working in agricultural sector. It was noted in the North American literature that female FSFWs are at increased risk of injuries due to improper machinery, equipment and tools use [7]. Among pregnant workers, increased incidences of pesticide and weedicide chemicals and veterinary pharmaceutical exposures had resulted in reproductive health concerns and miscarriages [7]. Studies in Canada and US among FSFWs have identified agrochemicals and heat exposure related illnesses, musculoskeletal injuries from repetitive motions, ubiquitous posture, resulting from manually lifting heavy loads, in addition to motor vehicle and machinery injuries [1]. Migrant farmers live in poor housing conditions in the host country and the researchers in Canada and US have noted unhealthy living and working environments, with the presence of mold, pesticide, weedicide residues, infested with disease carrying pests, rodents, mice and cockroaches in occupational and residential settings. Authors from a US study found a significant association between poor indoor living environments and upper respiratory symptoms among migrant farm workers [8]. Given these research-based evidence on farm workers tendency to be prone to illnesses and injuries and engagement in high risk occupations, occupational health and safety guidelines and procedures plays a critical role in this population. A section in this chapter will outline findings from a scoping review on existing guidelines lead by authors research group.

The living conditions and health and safety issues of FSFWs raise a global health and human rights issues. Stemming from research findings, many researchers share concerns on violation of human rights in access to sanitary conditions and denial of access to timely and needed healthcare. This vulnerable population shares common occupational health safety issues despite the country of origin and the host country of working. This chapter illustrates case studies and research conducted in one province in Canada, Nova Scotia, while elucidating the issues that are common to all migrant farm workers around the world that are stemming from the literature. Canada employs between 27,000and 42,000 foreign seasonal farm workers annually and United States employs around 3 million from Caribbean countries [9]. Of these positions, 1855 were in the province of Nova Scotia, where case studies were resonated [10]. Foreign seasonal farm workers come to Canada under the Seasonal Agricultural Workers Program (SAWP) and Temporary Foreign Worker Program (TFWP). SAWP workers come to Canada from Mexico and 11 Caribbean countries and can stay and work in Canada for up to 8 months [1]. Canada has a publicly funded universal healthcare system that covers necessary primary, secondary and tertiary healthcare with an exception of coverage for prescription medications, dental and vision care, physiotherapy and ambulance services, for all citizens, permanent residents and those who are on minimum of one-year work permit [11]. Whereas refugees and refugee claimants are covered by the Interim Federal Health program which covers almost all of the basic care [11]. Students are eligible for government health insurance after 1 year of residency in Canada. FSFWs do not fall into any of those Canadian healthcare eligibility categories due to their eight-month long contract obligations even if they return year after year for nearly 15 years. FSFWs contractual obligations dictate that the need to purchase private medical insurance, a portion of the cost is paid by the employee from hourly wages and the rest is covered by the employer [12].

1.1 Health and safety insurance coverage

The SAWP workers' contract stipulates that the workers are required to have health insurance and additional workers' compensation insurance coverage and transportation to medical facilities must be provided by the employers [13]. However, the reality of the situation requires further attention. Our research revealed contradictions to the written obligations, that are clearly stated in the contract documents. Wherein the employers' agreement states "*That according to the approved guidelines and regulations in the province/territory where the WORKER is employed the EMPLOYER shall take the WORKER to obtain health coverage in a timely manner.*" [13], which never becomes a reality since provincial regulations requires minimum of 12-month residency in the province of Nova Scotia and SAWP workers who comes for an eight-month contract never becomes eligible. New provisions have been added to the contract due to COVID-19, whereby the employer is required to submit a Housing Inspection Report prior to or during the time of application to Citizenship and Immigration Canada to obtain farm permits under SAWP (12). Workplace safety insurance in Canada is provided by provincial insurance provider Workers Compensations Board of Canada and the SAWP contract indicates that the employers must ensure that the workers are covered by provincial workplace safety insurance at no cost to them and in a situation that private insurance plan is preferred employers, must ensure the coverage is the same as the provincial plan [12].

1.2 Vulnerability

Only a few studies have examined the health and safety of SAWP in Canada and how the contractual obligations were met was understudied. The limited research has revealed significant barriers for healthcare accessibility, lack of proper occupational health and safety standards and noncompliance to existing guidelines. Recent global pandemic of COVID-19 has claimed three FSFW deaths and thousands of other FSFWs have been tested positive in Canada. There is an outcry from activist groups representing FSFWs, demanding actions on justice on migrant workers' health. This population falls under vulnerable populations based on Canadian public health guidelines. According to the Public Health Agency of Canada, vulnerable communities of COVID-19 includes those with; difficulties in communication, difficulties in accessing healthcare and engaging in preventive activities such as frequent hand washing, covering coughs and sneezes, difficulties in accessing transportation, unstable employment and working conditions, living in geographically isolated remote areas and insecure and inadequate housing conditions [14]. Albeit FSFWs have all of the above conditions that categorize them as vulnerable to COVID-19, there were no proper health safety measures taken to prevent their exposure to COVID-19.

This chapter comprise findings from three studies. Author led research team carried out a scoping reviews of the documents from non-governmental and governmental agencies, specifically aiming at the health and safety of FSFWs, followed by individual interviews with FSFWs and farmers (their employers). Third scoping review was carried out on COVID-19 related public health measures and extent to which these measures were applied to FSFWs in Canada using gray literature, pertaining to pandemic related health and safety concerns of the FSFWs. In this chapter, attention will be paid to contractual obligations of FSFWs through the documents available to them and the status of implementation of occupational health and safety guidelines will be examined through. Resurrection of occupational health and safety is a joint effort of the workers and employers. I have presented an exploration of present working conditions, individual and systemic barriers and incentives that prevent/promote hazardous working environments. Finally, existing guidelines and policies and the research-based evidence on individual and systemic factors that impede or promote occupational health and safety of FSFWs will be applied and evaluated to COVID-19 pandemic case scenario using the findings from the third scoping review. Given the limited geographical scope of the authors interview data, comparisons will be made to research findings that are stemming from other national and international research findings. This chapter will be finalized by making recommendations, on how to manage personal protective measures, implement policies and practices, focusing broadly on physical and mental health of FSFWs.

2. Occupational health and safety standards, guidelines, and policies

Foreign workers' legal residence status is tied to their employment contractual obligations, which stipulates access to healthcare, occupational health insurance, working and living conditions. Thus, individual workers lack full control over maintaining their own health and safety conditions, even if the guidelines are stipulated by the inter-governmental authorities of sending and receiving countries. The FSFWs' legal residence status in Canada is entirely based on their employment contractual stipulations that results in lack of control in determining their own health and safe working and living circumstances, since they are fully dependent on the conditions set by their employers [15–17]. The situation of lack of policies and regulations to protect foreign worker conditions is not unique to Canada. In Norway, though they have established different regulations for foreign seasonal workers, called transitional rules, the Norwegian researchers found these state-level formal labour regulations were not sufficiently implemented at the farm level resulting in structurally disempowered Polish farm workers, who had to accept the unhealthy working conditions provided by their Norwegian employers [18]. In Thailand, the existing regulations for local farm workers' protection from; labour, health, housing and sanitary conditions and health insurance, do not apply to migrant workers [19]. More so the existing policies, regulations and standards are not translated into accessible information. Canadian researchers have identified lack of information resources as a barrier to the maintenance of FSFWs health in Ontario, British Columbia, and Nova Scotia [15–17]. The situations of lack of proper labour regulations to protect migrant farm workers and evidence of non-compliance to existing guidelines were universal and were not unique to one country.

In the first scoping review, we reviewed 27 online documents including FSFW recruitment documents, contracts, and information provided by relevant non-governmental and governmental agencies, pertaining to occupational health and safety of migrant farm workers in Canada. Inductive analysis of the text data collected from the documents revealed (a) lack of clear identification of parties responsible for implementing and monitoring health and safety guidelines and (b) there were no mechanisms of facilitating existing health and safety information dissemination to FSFWs. Upon further review, it became clear that documents were not targeted specifically towards FSFWs and several documents were written at very high reading levels, at collage level and none of the FSFWs has reached that level. This "*passing the buck*" practice of evading the responsibility to keep FSFWs occupationally healthy and free from injuries needs to be fully explored.

2.1 Parties responsible for monitoring health and safety guidelines

The scoping review of the documents revealed that the health and safety of Canadian FSFWs is the joint effort of three parties: a) workers, b) employers, and/or c) third parties including federal health agencies, Canadian police, workers' home government organizations and agents, farm owners (where not the employer), and local, provincial, and Canadian labour and social development departments. Workers are responsible for helping employers to make the workplace safe by ensuring they obtain sufficient training to safely carry out their assigned tasks and refusing to carry out tasks they deem unsafe. Employers (farmers) are responsible for ensuring safety in the workplace by following provincial labour regulations and occupational health and safety guidelines. Third parties are responsible for monitoring the necessary guidelines and policies are followed by the two parties, workers and employers. None of the documents indicated, how the multi-partied responsibilities are imposed, implemented, monitored and assessed to ensure health and safety of FSSFWs. According to the government of Canada, Temporary Foreign workers your rights are protected document stated ""*All workers in Canada have the right to a safe workplace. Canada has laws to protect workers from unsafe working conditions. While some jobs may have more risk than others, no one should feel that the work they are doing is unsafe*." [13]. In reality, the protection of the rights are not facilitated, and the laws of protection are not conveyed. Even when they feel that the work is unsafe, there is no way out of the situation due to the fear of losing their job and denial of rehiring again. The international literature suggests two models of responsibilities related to Occupational Safety and Health of workers: (a) introspective model, the one which directs resources to the worker's need and (b) extrospective model is the one, which ensures safety standards prior to seeing the effect on workers [3, 4]. Given that FSFWs work in hazardous work environments, their risk of occupational injuries is high and the need to follow safety protocols should be made mandatory prior to seeing the need. Therefore, the extrospective model would be more appropriate.

2.2 Health and safety information dissemination

The shared responsible model for FSFWs workplace health and safety guidelines lack implementation strategies and therefore the level of outreach is questionable. All documents listed pertinent information about health and safety of FSFWs, the language used in each document was not necessarily targeted towards workers and there are no means to ensure the workers understand about occupational health and safety measures. Since the documents are not written at the level of their comprehension, it is unlikely the workers read them. Our research revealed that eighty-four percent of the English documents were written at a college level or greater and the two contracts that FSFWs workers are required to sign before coming to Canada are written at a college graduate level. Thus, while information and resources exist (although limited), it is questionable as to whether this information is finding its way into the hands of FSFWs. This echoes the findings of an Australian study, whereby the researchers found that there is a significant quantity of occupational health and safety resources that exist in Australia, though this information does not necessarily make it into the hands of workers, thus leaving migrant farm workers to rely on word-of-mouth information which may not be reliable [20]. Arguably, the existing health and safety regulations are there for marketing to attract FSFWs and for the purpose of branding the name of the host country in the international labour arena, not necessarily with an intention to keep the workers healthy and safe.

3. Occupational health issues: tri-partied perspectives

Agriculture related health issues has been categorized into eight categories; personal, psychosocial, farm, machinery, chemical, biological, and musculoskeletal [21]. In those categorizations, personal health issues are related to injuries from machinery and farm operations and the risk of those are associated with old age (fall and traumatic injuries), young age (machine operations) and chronic health conditions that impairs mobility. Stress has been noted as a major psychological illness and long hours and working alone in an isolated environment with less access to healthcare facilities put this population at increased risk for stress. Farm machinery related injuries are noted as resulting from old equipment and defective protective gear use as well as lack of safety labelling and protective structures on the machines [21]. Chemical and biological exposure related illnesses are primarily due to pesticide exposures and biological exposures are noted as from micro-organisms, viruses, toxins (from biological sources), spores, fungi, and bio-active substances that are a threat to human health [21]. A complete list of health issues of migrant farm workers in North America has been published and includes; musculoskeletal, ocular, dermatologic, psychological and sexual and reproductive health [22].

The author's research group conducted individual interviews using a semi-structured interview guide among three groups; FSFWs (sample size of eight), local seasonal farm workers (sample size of four) and farmers (sample size of six), who employed them in the province of Nova Scotia, Canada. This was a hard to reach population and snowball sampling method was used to find participants. Participating FSFWs were from Mexico and Jamaica and language difficulties were facilitated using both Spanish and English interviews. The age range of FSFWs was 33–52 years and the local farm workers were between 25 and 53 olds. The FSFWs all were married, and each have between 1 and 6 children, all of whom are living with their wives in their country of origin. Only 2 female local farmworkers were among the study participants. There were 25 different health conditions mentioned by the workers that can be categorized into two groups: work related physical environment issues such as aallergies, asthma, sun burns, eye irritations, skin conditions and sunstrokes; whereas occupational related Injuries included were; hernia, pain and soreness, slipped disk and tendonitis. Other illnesses noted were appendicitis, arthritis, blood pressure, dental problems, diabetes, encephalitis, flu, heart murmur, stomach cancer and ulcer. No psychological issues were reported, but the discussion eluded of work related stress, loneliness and missing home. The occupational health issues noted by the study participants fall into the categories noted in the literature for all agricultural workers [21] as well as migrant farm workers in Canada and elsewhere [22].

3.1 Occupational health and safety issues: Workers perspective

One of the perspectives that we uncovered in our interview data analysis was health issues emerging from lack of proper personal protective equipment. Besides one video, there were no other instructional detailed information releases on personal protective equipment use that we were able to identify. Personal protective equipment (PPE) to be used in the farms included in a video were: work gloves to prevent cuts, bruises and to protect from animals; hearing protectors to prevent noisy equipment use (more than 85 decibels), eye protectors (safety glasses), hard hats (depending on the type of work), steel toed boots to protect from heavy construction areas, reflective clothing to ensure visibility to protect from stuck by farm machinery, respirators and face masks to protect from pesticide and dust exposures and chemical safe overalls to protect from chemical exposures [23]. The English language instructional video further instructs to use sunscreen to prevent from skin burning, sunglasses and a sun hat. We have no evidence that FSFWs have watched any videos or any other paper-based instructions on this matter. However, availability of information from different sources are evident.

Our scoping review of the documents revealed that three parties are responsible for ensuring these personal safety and health protections from a safety standpoint [23]. FSFWs are responsible to ensure that they obtained necessary training to ensure workplace safety and some places have made the videos, posters and pamphlets available. Most of the information stand as optics to satisfy the government labour regulations but there are no assurance or mechanisms to ensure the information is actually reaching out to workers. The government of Canada seasonal agricultural worker program contract indicates that it is the responsibility of the worker to refuse to work in areas that deem unsafe. Employers are responsible for ensuring workplace safety and to follow labour regulations in their jurisdiction [12]. Our interview findings uncovered the reality.

According to one FSFW:

> *"And when I first got there, it was like in early May. I remember it was still really cold in Nova Scotia in May. Like it was often rainy and below like 12 degrees, so like everyone's hands were numb and there was no, no like [to protect my hands]. I sort of got the initial vibe of like toughen up, but like I have really bad blood circulation and like I just didn't have that problem in British Columbia [one of the warm weather provinces], because the temperature was just never that low where we were working."*

The above explanation indicates the status of protective equipment use. Even basic winter gloves to protect from frostbites were not used. One may argue that it is up to the worker to use them but if the use of protective equipment was made mandatory and monitored, the bad blood circulation would have been avoided. Another aspect that emerged from above statement was the intention of avoidance of PPE use was to be "*toughen up*", making themselves strong to the extent to make adaptation to cope up with the environment. Additional Personal protective equipment use was seen by workers as "*getting in the way*" to carry out the assigned tasks quickly. There were also incidents of knowing the need to use PPE, but without proper inspection from the authority or appropriate guard, they miss PPE use and then become prone to serious injuries. One participant explained an injury occurred in a corn field.

According to him; "*Yeah llike when I work in the corn field, we have goggles, we always have glasses on. One day I did not have glasses and a leaf probably whacked me in the eye when I was walking through the corn. It was bad and I had to go to the doctor and take time off.*"

This clearly indicates that this shared responsibility of PPE use was not implemented appropriately.

Participants reported exacerbation of existing chronic conditions, such as high blood pressure, diabetes and ulcer, but the doctors were attempting to use disease management using a life style change approach. This was something FSFWs noted as distinct from their country. They are used to getting treatment even for slightly elevated blood pressure and ulcers. They indicated that:

> *"Every day if I go to a doctor, doctor in Jamaica say, I must be sick, can't take it anymore, if I do not have blood pressure medication and my doctor will give me pills. So when I come up here and if I go to doctor here, if I don't have medication that I took from Jamaica there, they won't give me [prescriptions]. There [in Jamaica] for example there in there put in machine and my hand there and the blood pressure is saying one forty they give me pills. Here [in Canada] they say it is not too high."*

The author's research revealed undesirable work and living environments. They indicted that "*Working here is different from home. Even if it is raining you still have to work. Working seven days a week in rainfall and sunshine. Sun gets really, really hot you still have to be out there.*" However, according to the FSFWs' contract, employers are supposed to provide suitable accommodation and workers have the right to refuse the work deem unsafe [12]. The poor conditions of bunk house they live lead to exacerbation of asthma and respiratory conditions. As one FSFW noted:

> *"Conditions in bunkhouses were generally poor and often overcrowded…you get put in a house, and that was disgusting, cause that's not how we live in our country. Oh my god. Musty smelling. Like dogs, smells awful. Two to three guys in a little room, single beds. You got at least six or eight men in the bunkhouse."*

Occupational health issues are not limited to lack of PPE use and unhealthy work environments. Participants reported ergonomic conditions associated with repetitive and overuse of hands and knee problems for standing up for too long, back problems after being in the bending down posture for too long. Literature indicates the most prevalent exposure was related to repetitive movements and resulting illnesses that varied from carpel tunnel syndrome, knee, neck and shoulder issues and back problems due to spending prolong periods of bending down [22]. A study conducted in Ontario, Canada in 2003 interviewed Mexican and Caribbean workers, in their country after returning from Canada and they have indicated that they received proper training to handle machinery and chemicals but they were not given necessary protective equipment to wear [24]. As our study participants revealed those participants also expressed fear of reprisals if they report to authorities. One in five workers they interviewed reported ailments or injuries including vertebrae and knee problems, skin diseases, respiratory tract infections, hypertension, allergies and depression was reported among older workers [24]. Those conditions were similar to problems noted by our study participants.

Irrespective of stipulated work hours in the contract seasonal workers chose to work long hours, as long as 9–12 hours a day, for 6–7 days a week and inevitably they became prone to repetitive injuries and posture related ergonomic health conditions. Our study participants added knee problems resulting from standing up for 9–10 hours a day for 6–7 days a week. Attending primary care physician ordered tests and a specialist appointment was given after 8 months of the date of daignosis. As one worker said:

> *"Uh, da da da, they wanted to do a scope, last time I was talking to them and I need to wait to get down to a certain specialist in [name of town]. So I think that would've been back in January now. And they said it could be 8 months to a year before I can get down to see this gentleman."*

Given that the FSFWs are in the host country for 8 months only, leaving him to see the specialist is not realistic. One study participant indicated that he had to continue working, limping and no other treatment like physiotherapy nor aids such as knee pads were offered. This neglect of FSFW's work related injuries were common issue that some of the other study participants also revealed. This brings another dimension; racism, discrimination and neglect faced by FSFWs in accessing healthcare and offering solutions that are impractical while ignoring quick fix practical solutions to help patients falls into the realm of neglect.

Mental or emotional health issues were not reported among our study participants but expressions like "*missing home*" and "*home is a paradise*" were always mentioned. Our participants' conversations spring from missing home, family and independent lifestyles that they had in their country of origin. They often mentioned they are "*living for home*" or "*working for home*" and the living conditions, long hours and missing their family do not matter much. A study conducted among Mexican FSFWs to Canada indicated their expressions of anxiety and/

or mood disorders as "nerves" without medicalizing into a disease category [22]. Those research particiapnts explanation of feelings of missing home and loneliness is similar that we have observed among our study participants. When considering occupational health of FSFWs it is vital to pay attention to the symptoms of mental and emotional health without labelling since these conditions go undiagnosed or the workers try to hide to show them as able bodied or try to be "toughen up". There was a case of a memory loss of one of his bunk mates as reported by a study participant, presumably, due to an accident of hard object hitting his head or encephalitis. Wearing helmets was a foreign concept for these workers. He noted that his co-workers stayed in the hospital for a month and when he returned, he was unable to remember, where he was and what his friends' names were. The employer sent the worker home (back to the country of origin) upon returning from hospital. This type of injuries can be considered as permanent damages with lifelong disabilities and impairments. Apparently, the practice of sending the workers, who are ill and unable to carry out the work as per contract, called medical repatriation is a common practice and a study conducted in Ontario found there were 4.62% respirations due to medical reasons. Of those 41.3% were surgical related and 25.5% external injuries including poisoning reported during the study period 2001–2011 [25].

3.2 Occupational Health and safety issues of Canadian farm workers

All of the four (two females and two males) Canadian seasonal farm workers, who participated in the research lived outside of the farm and one worked part-time two days a week and the others work 6 days a week. They noted that their work hours are negotiated with the employer and they often get a 15-minute break before lunch, one-hour lunch break, another fifteen-minute break in the afternoon and "*leave home to make supper*". They have the negotiating power with the employer since they are protected by the Canadian labour regulations. FSFWs never mentioned about taking fifteen-minute breaks but taking half an hour for lunch. FSFWs intention was to put as many as hours possible during their short stay in Canada with the sole aim of "working for home", for feeding their family and for educating their children and they do not have the option of having unemployment insurance for the rest of the year that they are not working, like Canadian farm workers do. A scoping review conducted on published research among Canadian temporary foreign workers concluded that their health issues are resulting from precarious immigrant status [26]. This precarious immigrant status is a real threat to their occupational health. Though repetitive injuries, aches and pains may be common to all farm workers, inevitably Canadian farm workers are more educated on health and safety regulations and PPE use than FSFWs, who face language and accessibility barriers. It was also revealed in our research that Canadian farmers are accustomed to take over the counter medications, pain killers and personal protective gear such as sun protectors, goggles, kneecaps and gloves.

3.3 Occupational Health and safety issues of FSFWs: employers perspectives

Two different opinions about occupational health of FSFWs were uncovered, when compared with FSFWs ideas about issues and Canadian farmers (employers) sentiments about their foreign employees' health issues. Some farmers mentioned the workers as "whinny", those who take minor illnesses, like muscle sore, cuts and bruises that general Canadians would ignore, as serious. Farmers further explained the reason for being concerned about minor illnesses as major, because "*their physical health is their bread and butter*". Following two quotes from two farmers supports these perspectives.

"We always do incident reports. But there's never anything serious. It just seemed like one might've had like uh tingling in his foot or something just really odd [minor complain]. And something that that the typical Canadian would ignore. Like they say the typical North American man acts like he's dying when he just has a cold, but then if he's really dying, he ignores it and then it's always too late. But those guys would complain, where a lot of Canadian guys will just shrug that off. One of our guys, one of our local people had a stroke here at work and he ignored it and he thought he hurt his arm trimming cabbage."

Farmers were also under the impression that "*they [FSFWs] are thinking oh you know well there's a health care system here that's free and everything and then I want to take advantage of it. Healthcare is not free* [in their country]," and when in Canada, a portion of insurance cost is deducted from their hourly wages. It is mandatory for them to have private health insurance and a portion is also paid by the employer. The notion of FSFWs as complainants of minor illness that the Canadians would shrug off was consistent with all of the farmers that we interviewed. One of the facts that sprung out of farmer's description of workers' occupational injuries, was farmers never paid attention to the fact that those injuries would have been avoided if the workers were wearing protective equipment or if they were given training on correct posture and maneuvering. For example, one farmers explained an eye injury that could have been avoided if the worker was wearing goggles or safety glasses as follows.

"He was picking roots and he was tugging on a root like that, and the root let go and went up here and hit him in the corner of the eye. So you know, he got some dirt in his eye and stuff and the farmer's wife took him out patients clinic and they flushed his eye out and stuff, put a little patch over it and they [healthcare providers] told him he would he definitely gonna live and go back home fine."

However, serious incidents such of breaking two ribs after falling from a moving wagon was reported by the farmer as the fault of the worker since he was sitting on a pole, something he was not supposed to do. There was no other safe sitting arrangement (seat with a belt to have buckled up) in the wagon. Had the worker have received proper training and safety instructions, on riding on a wagon safely, the injury would have been avoided. However, the following description indicates that the fault was always on the worker and farmer took this serious debilitating injury very lightly. Safety instructions should have been given prior to assigning the tasks.

"Another fella he was actually doing what he wasn't supposed to be doing and he knew he wasn't supposed to be doing it but. He was standing on the pole of the wagon when they were gathering up irrigation pipes, he slipped off the pole and hit the arm on the tractor, kind of caught him underneath the rib here, and I think it cracked two ribs or something. And they taped him all up and you know and he I think he was off a week or something."

There were serious incidents of diagnosis of encephalitis, exacerbation of chronic conditions such as high blood pressure among FSFWs, diabetes, ulcers, and hernia that the farmers reported. Chronic conditions such as diabetes and ulcers may not have direct links farm work related occupational health issues. But work-related stress and poor eating habits can have indirect impacts on diabetes and ulcers. There is literature suggesting high prevalence of hernia in males engaged in manual labour. Encephalitis is known to be associated with tick bites and one worker, who contacted encephalitis was left with a lifetime disability of memory loss. As one farmer indicated the worker who contacted encephalitis was young, tall healthy looking Mexican and he was confused in the first week of arrival. Upon admission to the hospital his condition deteriorated so fast he was in a medically induced coma. Mexican government flew his wife over and he was in the hospital for the whole season. The employer washed his hands off by saying "*well that as soon as he was in the accident* [ward], *we didn't see him anymore and we didn't deal with it at all. It was just it was all the governments* [Mexican and Canadian] *and the medical system, the ambulances and then and right away his liaison service had to get involved. We did go down to visit him a couple times and so*." No investigation was carried out how he contacted encephalitis and how his family survived without him sending money and how they are surviving with a permanent debilitating condition afterwards.

Interview data revealed that the employers treated FSFWs seeking treatment for occupational related injuries as "*whinny*", "*those who take advantage of the healthcare system*" and "*seeking treatment for minor ailments that Canadians would shrug off*", within which even serious injuries were considered as the fault of the worker. There is an outcry of mass media in the past about medical repatriation, that seriously ill workers are sent back to their country without treating in Canada. Canadian researchers indicated that the employers lack of empathy lead to vision loss of a worker who sprayed pesticide accidently on his eyes and he was not allowed to have a shower and ultimately the worker was medically repatriated. He was not given any compensation since he did not know how to maneuver the governance system [27]. Some NGO representing workers' rights have questioned lack of bargaining power to represent FSFWs rights and privileges. A systematic review conducted among studies on Canadian temporary foreign workers in the agricultural sector included the similar health issues reported by our study participants, mental health, poor housing and sanitation and they also noted language barriers in accessing healthcare all shaped by the precarious immigrant status in Canada [24].

Our research revealed one farm that is out of ordinary, farmers cared about the occupational health and safety of workers. This farm is run by a young university educated couple. According to the male owner as a rule, the workers break off around lunch time and then rest until the sun set, at 4:00 pm, to avoid sun burns and heat strokes. He mentioned about two people dying of heat stroke in the past. Another farmer said if a FSFW is sick he tried to give them time off or assign light duties to him and "*if they can't work there is no expectation from the farmer they should work*." He further iterated they have developed a culture that they do not want anybody to get hurt. The second farmer further iterated that the FSFWs are well experienced and some of them come for many years to the same farm and they do understand what is safe and what is unsafe.

4. COVID-19 public health measures – testing, isolation, social distancing and contract tracing

The primary focus of this section of the chapter is on the provision of evaluation of barriers and challenges to meet the government regulated public health standards-personal protective measures of infection control for COVID-19, focusing on living and working conditions of FSFWs that uncovered in aforementioned research findings. I was unable to find published scientific research findings on this population on the topic of COVID-19. This section covers findings from a scoping review of gray literature and government documents, as a starting point for further scientific explorations. According to the advocacy group Justice for Migrant Workers more than 1000 Canadian migrant agricultural workers have been diagnosed with COVID-19 and three deaths were reported among them [28]. Canadian government opened boarders for FSFWs as a response to an outcry from farmers across Canada indicating billions of dollars will be lost in the food production sector due to labour shortage. The Canadian government has developed regulatory conditions that included a safety measures of mandatory house inspection and a report obtained within the past three years has to be submitted by the employer at the time of application or else with an agreement to submit an updated inspection report within the duration of FSFWs employment [29]. There was a link in the document to the letter provided by the minister of health that gives other mandatory public health measures such as 14-day quarantine requirement, with self-isolation, accommodation allowing social distancing of 2 meters apart, providing materials for adequate sanitation and cleaning and disinfecting surfaces regularly [29]. Our previous research indicated that pre-COVID health and safety measures never reached the workers, not written at a format and a linguistic level of comprehension of the workers. We have evidence from the scoping review of COVID-19 incidents reports that the new public health measures were also limited to inaccessible printed materials and never reached a state of full capacity implementation. No monitoring was provided in some cases and when complains were launched about farmers the government lead inquiries were not independent and unbiased. The following description were revealed from the brief scoping review.

The scoping review revealed reports of non-compliance to public health measures. It was said that "*upon the worker's arrival, the government has gone on to take little responsibility for the health and safety of migrant workers. This has allowed for an increase in migrant worker abuse and the spread of several outbreaks within migrant populations*."

The form of abuse and neglect that dated few years back had continued throughout up to the pandemic taking different forms. It was reported that "*Between 2009 and 2018, 3100 complaints were submitted by Mexican workers to the Mexican Ministry of Labour on the issues they faced on Canadian farms, reporting frequent instances of worker abuse, rat-infested dormitories, sewage issues, and gas leaks.*" [30], all of which had happened within the last 3-year period. It is unclear that if the housing inspection report was submitted within the three-year period that granted migrant workers to be employed and if so how those critical public health threats were not detected during the inspection. Perhaps the answer is related to the following report. Workers who were in quarantine in un-health living environments had complained through migrant right activists and the "government agent" informed the supervisor of the farm about an upcoming inspection and they said "*that a supervisor on the farm chose four employees to speak to the agent. The supervisor told the workers to say they were being treated well, that they were being paid OK, even though they weren't, and that if they don't communicate these things to the government agent, that they're going to be deported and they'll never work here (as part of) the program again*." [31]. Many researchers had pointed out the precarious immigrant status had created diminished power for change and demand for rights for FSFWs. There were also reports of noncompliance to social distancing, when quarantined up to 40 migrant workers in a large bunk house and they had to share the same bathroom [30]. According to work the living conditions had made it impossible not to spread the virus.

Pandemic brought new dimensions of abuse and neglect due to mandatory confinement regulated by the government. As one document (30) reported a statement of a FSFW:

> *Some farm owners have threatened to fire workers for leaving bunkhouses during quarantine while others have refused to allow migrant workers to leave or to allow visitors to come onto the farm property throughout the pandemic. One worker recounts a farmer telling him, "If you set one foot off the farm, I'll be the first one to call the cops."*

International Labour Organization has given very limited attention to migrant farm workers working conditions, in terms of enforcing legislature to safeguard temporary foreign workers' occupational health and safety, in addition, the host country legislature is poorly applicable to this vulnerable population of workers due to their nature of temporariness and precariousness [32]. My scoping review findings supports that existing situations of neglect and abuse of FSFWs occupational health issues has further exacerbated due to COVID-19 related public health control measures as one NGO participant summed up ""*Because we do not have proper rights, they step on our necks*," [28].

5. Limitations for generalizability

This chapter consisted of findings from three different types of analytical studies, one of which consisted of analysis of online resources available to farmers and workers, the second study brought forward farmers' perspectives, obtained from personal interviews with them; both were conducted according tri-council guidelines after approving by the Dalhousie University Health Sciences ethics review board. Our interview data collection and analysis assured scientific rigor and the research team included three university professors: an experienced qualitative researcher, Canadian occupational health expert researcher and an immigrant health research expert. Findings from the third study, a scoping review of COVID-19 associated health risks for FSFWs were analyzed using online government documents and reports from media investigations. It is customary that media tend to draw attention to negative incidents to raise awareness among authorities. Without carrying out national inventory of all farm related occupational illnesses and injury, generalizability of findings is not warranted. There were common health and justice issues that came from published research on migrant farm workers in Canada and in other geographies that warrant further attention. Even barriers related PPE use and lack of knowledge and training on safe working practices were common across different geographies, nationally and globally.

6. Recommendations for improvement: farmers and workers suggestions

Farmers were under the impression that there is always room for improvement. One of the suggestions made was having physiotherapist and massage therapist to train the workers. One farmer put this as:

> *"Well one thing I've been thinking about on our own farm and maybe in other farms it might apply, or the program in general but give given that a lot of the work the guys do is kind of repetitive motions and things like that. And I was thinking like the physiotherapists or [ergonomist] who can train people you know on good posture and showing them certain exercises you can do every hour or so to sort of you know do minimize carpal tunnel and you know things [repetitive motion injuries] like that."*

Another farmer suggested rotating workers on the same task, within one work shift to avoid repetitive injuries and also to reduce stress of engaging in the task. Another obvious recommendation was to provide training to avoid ergonomic and posture related injuries. According to one farmer:

> *"I'd like to try to get some of that in place, 'cause they you know they, a lot of the work is repetitive physical work and I mean rotating if there's a crew and there's*

> *different functions, so the guys kind of rotate through the day to the different positions so the, whatever the motions are they're doing, kind of changes to give the body a chance to recuperate and not get in to repetitive stress, tight syndromes uh muscle stress or whatever. So that that that's one thing there, I'd like to see."*

Another farmer suggested to have a fact sheet written in simple language. Farmers felt the need to support the workers to be healthy and to avoid occupational related injuries.

FSFWs also made suggestions for improvements. One suggestion was to have easy to understand safety training materials to be developed. For example, cartoon like characters to get the messages across to carry out tasks safely and provided an example of Mickey mouse using the rake and also to train them how to safely sharpen the tools and proper ways to kneel and stretch. A study conducted in Canada in the year 2003 interviewed FSFWs in their country of origin, after returning from their work term in Canada. They recommended to continue health insurance that they purchased while working in Canada, after they returned home enabling them to get the necessary treatments for the ailments and injuries that occurred while working in Canada [24].

7. Conclusions

In summary, this chapter provided an overview of foreign seasonal farmworkers occupational health and safety standards, incidences, and caveats to implementation of policies and regulations. While each author provided compelling and empirically rich observations based on local fields of study, generally lacking are broader global connections and policy discussions about how the problems raised can be meaningfully addressed. Following is a summary of findings.

- Occupational health and safety of this population is regulated as a tri-partied responsibility; of workers, of employers (farmers) and of non-governmental agencies and therefore none takes the full responsibility to implement existing guidelines and policies.

- There are no mechanisms to ensure the information is reaching out to the workers, albeit to the fact that the readability of the available information is written in a language at a level higher than workers level of education.

- In comparison with the limited data collected from Canadian farm workers, made it clear that FSFWs lack negotiating power to shape systemic changes to curb barriers to occupational health due to their precarious immigrant status of "working for home" and thus by putting long hours and days.

- Foreign seasonal farm workers arrive in Canada healthy, due to the pre migration screening procedures that allows only healthy immigrants to migrate, a well documented notion called "Health immigrant effect" [26]. This research revealed incidence of exacerbation of existing chronic conditions related poor work and eating habits that they continued after migrating to Canada.

- We have noted several forms of neglect and abuse, in accessing and promoting healthcare when needed, ignoring hazardous work environments and not providing proper training and safety equipment and neglecting basic public health and sanitary conditions. The forms of neglect of health issues resonated from farmers' (employer's) opinion about their workers in general as "whinny" and seeking treatments for minor ailments that a typical Canadian would ignore as well as their idea of FSFWs trying to take advantage of the healthcare that are "free", after buying private insurance. Neglect and abuse are interconnected. The form of abuse varies from minor issues such as allowing them to work without taking breaks in harsh weather conditions to serious actions of not allowing the worker to take a shower when toxic materials are sprayed on his eyes by an accident, an incident noted in the literature. COVID-19 related public health controlling measures were imposed in a manner that violated fundamental rights and privileges of this population of workers.

- **It is recommended** that there should be monitoring of tri-partied contract obligations, policies and practices are implemented appropriately and reaching to the workers in a manner (language and mode of dissemination) that is reachable to the foreign seasonal farm workers.

- **It is recommended** that farmers should be educated to change their attitude towards workers health related complains to consider them seriously enough to bring to medical attention.

- **It is recommended** there should policies and legislature in place to investigate serious incidents that requires medical repatriation to serve justice to the parties responsible.

- **It is recommended** to investigate medical repatriation by a third party and compensation scheme should be set up for life long debilitating injuries and occupational illnesses.

- **It is recommended** to establish a third party responsible for investigating neglect and abuse related complains.

Author details

Swarna Weerasinghe
Department of Community Health and Epidemiology, Dalhousie University, Halifax, Nova Scotia, Canada

*Address all correspondence to: swarna.weerasinghe@dal.ca

References

[1] Cole DC, McLaughlin JE, Hennebry JL, Tew MA. Precarious patients: Health professionals' perspectives on providing care to Mexican and Jamaican migrants in Canada's seasonal agricultural worker program. Rural and Remote Health. 2019;**19**:4

[2] Frank AL, McKnight R, Kirkhorn SR, Gunderson P. Issues of agricultural safety and health. Annual Review of Public Health. 2004;**25**:225-245

[3] Alho R, Helander MFOREIGNSEASONAL. FARM WORKERS' STRATEGIES AT THE MARGINS OF THE FINNISH WELFARE STATE: Informal networks and weak ties. Nordic Journal of Migration Research. 2016 Sep;**6**(3):148-157

[4] Caxaj CS, Cohen A. I will not leave my body here{"}: Migrant farmworkers" Health and safety amidst a climate of coercion. International Journal of Environmental Research and Public Health. 2019 Aug;**16**(15)

[5] Moyce SC, Schenker M. Migrant Workers and Their Occupational Health and Safety. In: Fielding, JE and Brownson, RC and Green, LW, editor. ANNUAL REVIEW OF PUBLIC HEALTH, VOL 39. 2018. p. 351-65. (Annual Review of Public Health; vol. 39).

[6] Earle-Richardson G, Jenkins PL, Slingerland DT, Mason C, Miles M, May JJ. Occupational injury and illness among migrant and seasonal farmworkers in New York state and Pennsylvania, 1997-1999: Pilot study of a new surveillance method. American Journal of Industrial Medicine. 2003 Jul;**44**(1):37-45

[7] Ramos AK, Girdziute L, Staric J, Rautianinen RH. Identifying vulnerable agricultural populations{"} at risk for occupational injuries and illnesses": A European perspective. Journal of Agromedicine.

[8] Kearney GD, Chatterjee AB, Talton J, Chen H, Quandt SA, Summers P, et al. The Association of Respiratory Symptoms and Indoor Housing Conditions among Migrant Farmworkers in eastern North Carolina. Journal of Agromedicine. 2014 Oct;**19**(4):395-405

[9] Employment and Social Development Canada. Annual Labour Market Impact Assessment Statistics 2008-2015 Primary Agriculture Stream [Internet]. 2016 [cited 2020 Aug 5]. Available from: https://www.canada.ca/en/employment-social- development/services/foreign-workers/reports/2014/lmia-annual- statistics/agricultural.html

[10] Employment and Social Development Canada. Temporary Foreign Worker Program [Internet]. 2020 [cited 2020 Aug 5]. Available from: https://www.canada.ca/en/employment-social-development/services/foreign-workers.html

[11] Government of Canada. Healthcare in Canada [Internet]. 2017 [cited 2020 Aug 5]. Available from: https://www.canada.ca/en/immigration-refugees-citizenship/services/new-immigrants/new-life-canada/health-care-card.html#:~:text=Canada's universal health-care system,for most health-care services.&text=All provinces and territories will,have a government

[12] Government of Canada. Contract for the Employment in Canada of Commonwealth Caribbean Seasonal Agricultural Workers - 2020 [Internet]. 2020 [cited 2020 Aug 5]. Available from: https://www.canada.ca/en/employment-social-development/services/foreign-workers/agricultural/seasonal-agricultural/apply/caribbean.html#h2.6

[13] Emplyment and Social Development Canada. Hire a Temporary Worker through the Seasonal Agricultural Worker Program: Program Requirements [Internet]. 2020 [cited 2020 Aug 5]. Available from: https://www.canada.ca/en/employment-social-development/services/foreign-workers/agricultural/seasonal-agricultural/requirements.html

[14] Public Health Agency of Canada. CORONAVIRUS DISEASE (COVID-19) VULNERABLE POPULATIONS AND COVID-19 [Internet]. 2020 [cited 2020 Aug 7]. Available from: https://www.canada.ca/content/dam/phac-aspc/documents/services/publications/diseases-conditions/coronavirus/covid-19-vulnerable-populations/update-covid-19-vulnerable-populations-eng.pdf

[15] Hennebry J, Preibisch K, Mclaughlin J. Health across Borders-Health Status, Risks and Care among Transnational Migrant Farm Workers in Ontario. 2012.

[16] Otero G, Preibisch K. Farmworker Health and Safety: Challenges for British Columbia. WorkSafeBC [Internet]. 2010 [cited 2020 Aug 12];1-103. Available from: https://www.deslibris.ca/ID/229186

[17] Brantford L, Mclaughlin J. Falling through the Cracks: Seasonal Foreign Farm Workers' Health and Compensation across Borders [Internet]. Vol. 21, The IAVGO Reporting Service. 2007 [cited 2020 Aug 12]. Available from: http://scholars.wlu.ca/brantford_hshttp://scholars.wlu.ca/brantford_hs/2

[18] Rye JF, Andrzejewska J. The structural disempowerment of eastern European migrant farm workers in Norwegian agriculture. Journal of Rural Studies. 2010 Jan;**26**(1):41-51

[19] Thetkathuek A, Meepradit P, Sa-ngiamsak T. A cross-sectional study of musculoskeletal symptoms and risk factors in Cambodian fruit farm Workers in Eastern Region, Thailand. Safety and Health at Work. 2018 Jun;**9**(2):192-202

[20] Underhill E, Rimmer M. Itinerant foreign harvest workers in Australia: The impact of precarious employment on occupational safety and health. POLICY Pract Heal Saf. 2015;**13**(2):25-46

[21] Chattha HS, Corscadden KW, Zaman QU. Hazard identification and risk assessment for improving farm safety on Canadian farms. Journal of Agricultural Safety and Health. 2017 Jul;**23**(3):155-174

[22] Pysklywec M, McLaughlin J, Tew M, Haines T. Doctors within borders: Meeting the health care needs of migrant farm workers in Canada. Canadian Medical Association Journal. 2011 Jun;**183**(9):1039-1043

[23] Canadian Agricultural Safety Association. Foreign Worker Farm Safety Training Video – Canadian Agricultural Safety Association [Internet]. [cited 2020 Aug 26]. Available from: https://www.casa-acsa.ca/en/safetyshop-library/foreign-worker-farm-safety-training-video/

[24] The North-South Institute. A Review of the Canadian Seasonal Agricultural Workers Program Policy Brief Migrant Workers in Canada: Migrant Workers in Canada [Internet]. 2006 [cited 2020 Aug 29]. Available from: http://www.nsi-ins.ca/wp-content/uploads/2012/10/2006-Migrant-Workers-in-Canada-A-review-of-the-Canadian-Seasonal-Agricultural-Workers-Program.pdf

[25] Mysyk A, England M, Avila Gallegos JA. Nerves as embodied metaphor in the Canada/Mexico seasonal agricultural workers program. Medical Anthropology. 2008;**27**(4):383-404

[26] Salami B, Meharali S, Salami A. The health of temporary foreign workers in Canada: A scoping review. Can J PUBLIC Heal Can SANTE PUBLIQUE. 2015;**106**(8):E546-E554

[27] McLaughlin J. Falling through the Cracks: Seasonal Foreign Farm Workers' Health and Compensation across Borders. Heal Stud [Internet]. 2007 Oct 1 [cited 2020 Aug 28]; Available from: https://scholars.wlu.ca/brantford_hs/2

[28] Bogart N. Ontario sees jump in COVID-19 cases among farm workers | CTV News. CTV news [Internet]. 2020 [cited 2020 Aug 28]; Available from: https://www.ctvnews.ca/health/coronavirus/advocates-demand-ontario-shut-down-farms-as-covid-19-cases-soar-among-workers-1.5004897

[29] Emplymnet and Social Development Canada. Temporary Foreign Worker Program – COVID-19 - Canada.ca [Internet]. Government of Canada. 2020 [cited 2020 Aug 28]. Available from: https://www.canada.ca/en/employment-social-development/services/foreign-workers/notice-covid-19.html

[30] Gatehouse J. How undocumented migrant workers are slipping through Ontario's COVID-19 net | CBC News [Internet]. CBC investigation. 2020 [cited 2020 Aug 28]. Available from: https://www.cbc.ca/news/canada/leamington-migrant-workers-1.5633032

[31] Ziafati N. Migrant workers complain of conditions, threat of deportation on Nova Scotia farm | The Star [Internet]. The Star. 2020 [cited 2020 Aug 28]. Available from: https://www.thestar.com/news/canada/2020/08/01/migrant-workers-complain-of-conditions-threat-of-deportation-on-nova-scotia-farm.html

[32] McLaughlin J, Weiler AM. Migrant agricultural Workers in Local and Global Contexts: Toward a better life? Journal of Agrarian Change. 2017 Jul;**17**(3):630-638

Chapter 4

A Review of Ergonomic Evaluation of Occupational Hazard of Indian Agriculture Farm and Allied Activities

Surendra Prasad Tripathi, Surya Pratap Singh Somvanshi, Shyam Ranjan Kumar Singh and Anupam Mishra

Abstract

Women in India are the major workforce in agriculture and perform almost all the agricultural activities. Women constitute 25.51% of the total work force in the country. The rural women play a vital role in agriculture and other agro based processing activities. They spent more time on post-harvest activities than those pre-harvest activities. Environmental and occupational health issues among agricultural workers expressed high levels of concern about working in hot weather, agricultural injuries, pesticides, awkward posture and drudgery prone activities. User Eco-friendly tools can increase the working efficiency and reduce the working load health hazards on farm activities during agricultural activities.

Keywords: Agriculture Activities, musculoskeletal Problem, drudgery, health, work Load, women Participation, postural discomfort

1. Introduction

Women comprise approximately 25.51% of the total work force in India as per [1], of which approximately 18.5% and 24.9% are agricultural labourers and cultivators respectively while 47.5% work in household and other important agriculture-aiding fields. Women fulfill many crucial roles in the farming sectors, all the way from being general farmers to farming-entrepreneurs [2]. It was observed that more than 75 per cent women are involved in activities like winnowing, weeding, grading, threshing and cleaning of field farm operations [3]. If women were to be given the same opportunities in utilizing resources as men, the UN Food and Agriculture Organization estimates a rise in yields by up to 30%, which could have a chain effect by which a rise in total agricultural output by 4% is predicted along with reduction of the general hunger in population by 12–17%, which is about 100 million people [4]. The participation of farm women in agricultural activities suffer both by nature wise and extent wise by multiple of things including, local dimension in nature of labor, socio-economic strata of the farm families, ancestral family customs, change in nature of activities thanks to mechanization, introduction of your time and labour saving implements and ever changing nature of agro-climatic conditions [5].

Ergonomics is a multidisciplinary science that activities to make a better fit between the work and the worker to ensure their healthiness and well-being. It emphasizes on designing and arranging things so that workers can use them easily and safely. The International Ergonomics Association [6] defined ergonomics as a science that deals with understanding the interaction between humans and other elements of a socio-technical system. Using ergonomics in agriculture helps in reducing and removing the risks involved in work, machines, vehicles and the work environment which includes tools and materials, method of work, ambient conditions, physical environment and organization of work. Ergonomics and sustainable agriculture should go hand in hand with each other. Women contribute in overall farm production--average contribution--is estimated to be in the range of 60 to 65 percent of the total labour and in certain areas, the same contribution is even higher in percentages. Unfortunately even today, agriculture related activities rank as one of the most hazardous activities as it relies mostly on manual labour and people working in the fields of agriculture are exposed to a multiple varieties of hazards that are extremely damaging to their physical condition and well-being. People from rural communities and background often lack orientation and knowledge on the health related issues that they face. Farmwomen consider pain as a traditional part of work or let us say their *Karma* and seek medical assistance when the condition becomes ruthless or disabling. This same issue carries over to preventive measures designed to reduce the incidence of musculoskeletal injuries or other hazardous work exposures [7]. It was reported by [8] that the share of women labour force in agricultural operations is expected to be 55 percent by 2025 A.D. They participate in several farm operations putting many hours of productive manual labor daily. It is duly reported [9] that women contribute to plentiful responsibilities to undertake extensive range of duties both in the home and outside but their partaking is considered insignificant by the social order. They are at length involved in a variety of farm operations like transplanting, weeding, harvesting, processing, marketing and selling of food grains, fruits and vegetables etc. These activities not only require substantial time and energy but also are the sources of tremendous amount of drudgery. Drudgery, which is largely, envisaged as physical and mental damage, anguish, repetitiveness and hardship that are experienced by farmwomen while performing these farm operations. The drudgery prone situations lead to an assortment of health and mechanical hazards, which creates physical exhaustion fatigue and low productivity.

2. Methodology

The objective of seeking for recent articles related to ergonomic evaluation of occupational hazard of Indian agriculture farm and allied activities the common search engines of Google Scholar, Scopus PubMed and Science Direct were used. Once we were identifying a study, we made a methodical survey within the web site of the journal during which the study was published with the intention of detecting further studies. All the co-authors discussed on the content of the chosen papers and a few of them were excluded, because they did not meet a minimum of one among the inclusion criteria described below. Evaluating the methodology of the selected studies is a key step in carrying out and interpreting systematic literature reviews related to objective of study. Moreover, the literatures, reports and documents associated with this study are reviewed because the references to testify the knowledge we obtained and selected up.

While collecting the data; particular attention was given to the selection of respondent on physical fitness and prevalence of any serious health hazard. The anthropometer and weighing balance were used to measure the physical characteristics like height and weight. The grading of health status of women was done based on Body Mass Index. The BMI scores were interpreted as per the classification given by [10]. Stopwatch was used for recording the time determined for the farm women. The heart rate was recorded by using the heart rate monitor sphygmomanometer (Digital), based on the heart rate records, the following parameters were calculated. The results were statistically analyzed using test of significance (t- test at 5% level of probability) and simple regression (r) by the method proposed by [11]. For calculation of Energy Expenditure Rate from heart rate [12]. The cardiac cost of work is the total number of heart beats spent about the resting level in order to perform the work, The cardiac cost of revitalization is the total number of heart beats above the resting level occurring at the termination of work and return to the pre activity state [13].

1. Average heart rate during rest and work. Measured by (Digital) sphygmomanometer.

2. The energy expenditure per minute was estimated from the heart rate with the help of formula Energy expenditure (kJ/min) = (0.0114 x WHR – 0.68) 20.93

3. ΔHR (beats/min) = Average working heart rate – average heart rate during rest

4. Output (Kg/h) = yield/average time

5. Physiological cost reduction (%) = T^1 (ΔHR/Output) – T^2 (ΔHR/Output) x 100/ T^1

6. Cardiac cost reduction (%) = (CCW T^1- CCW T^2) x 100/ CCW T^1

The prevalence of musculoskeletal problems among agricultural workers were found using Psychophysical techniques developed by [14] 'Body Map' technique was used to determine musculoskeletal problems and Body Part Discomfort Score (BPDS) and Visual Analogue Discomfort (VAD) scale was used to assess Overall Discomfort Score (ODR) of the respondents while performing different agricultural activities. Taken as a whole, the Visual Analogue Discomfort (VAD) Scale was also employed to determine this discomfort score, which ranges from 0 to 10 for determining the level of discomfort with 10 being the highest level of while 0 indicating none. This tool emphasizes discomfort and not necessarily the pain felt. Since this method follows a ten-point scale, it is also more suitable for Indian workers due to ease of understanding. Discomfort Rating Scale 0: No discomfort 1–3: Light discomfort <3–5: Moderate discomfort <5–7: More than moderate discomfort <7–9: High discomfort <9–10: Extreme discomfort.

3. Extent of participation of women in agriculture farm and allied activities

Nature and extent of the involvement of women folk vary significantly from one region to another and even within a region. They take part largely in as many as 11 family operations out of total 17. While ploughing remains much male-dominated, women heavily involve themselves in activities like sowing/transplanting (86%), weeding (84%), storage of grains (78%), land preparation (72%), cleaning seeds for sowing (70%), gap filling (68%), manure and fertilizer application (68%), harvesting (64%), threshing and winnowing (62%) and rat control practices (58%) [15]. For the period of peak season of agriculture especially during harvesting time, women of farm families labor on an average seven to eight hours a day in the field. This is besides their everyday duties of cooking, fetching water, cleaning etc. [16]. Women are most active in areas like fertilizing, sowing, grain cleaning, drying, etc. Women also partake in almost all aspects of animal husbandry from collecting fodder and feeding the animals to collecting milk and disposing dunk [17].

4. Ergonomic evaluation of agriculture farm and allied activities

Relationship between Anthropometric measurements of women and work efficiency in an Indian context, ergonomic point of view, average age was found 33.39 ± 7.57 years, height 154.94 ± 3.61 cm and weight 51.33 ± 4.06 kg respectively. The mean Body Mass Index (BMI) was calculated using standard formula Weight in kilograms/ (Height in meters)^2 it was 21.39 ± 1.42 which meant that they were in the normal category during groundnut shelling for energy expenditure during the shelling by decorticator calculated 9.31 kJ/min in traditional practices, while by improved practice it was 18.94 kJ/min [18]. Anthropometric parameters studied by [19] female workers of different ages to assess the work methods and postural demands during work performance to enhance the operability, safety, convenience and comfort while performing domestic and occupational tasks [20]. The study showed that Vo2 max of the chosen women folk range from 16.1 to 64.8 ml/min with a mean value of 39.89 ml/min. and half of the respondents (50%) had very good physical fitness in the range of 41–45 ml/min. According to [21], the range of average heart rate lies between 153 and 180 beats/min. Nevertheless, the amount considered as a fair amount of work when considering a large sample of cardiac responses was below 130beats/min. The rates however ranged at 153.3/min for water-lifting and 140.3/min for pedal-threshing. Relatively, the increase in uptake of oxygen to workload ranged at 5–7% per 10 beats/min increase, with oxygen-pulse ratio being at various levels 43:120, 55:130, 61:140, and 74:150 [21]. The authors go on to say that stationing the oxygen intake, 120–132 beats/min can be achieved which signifies an average workload. Overall, energy expended throughout the day amongst people working in agriculture ranged (in MJ) between 10.3 to 11.7, of this number, 5.6 to 6.6 MJ (or between 53 and 56%) was used in a work day. The time-weighted average of the entire day comes to 7.2–8.1 kg/min. This implies that the comparatively, the load amounted only to around 20.22% of maximum oxygen uptake. However, if only the energy spent in a working day is considered, the time-weighted average was between 10.9–14.6 kg/min or 30–40% of maximum oxygen uptake.

4.1 Physiological parameters and energy expenditure

Generally, pulse is employed as an ergonomic measure to gauge the physiological or functional demands of labor on the individual workers [22]. The physiological point of view, the work demand or workload refers to the stress placed on the cardio-respiratory system and is decided by the energy cost and cardiac cost of work [23]. [18] reported physiological cost of work and energy expenditure in terms of heart rate were observed to be lower while performing selected activities with groundnut decorticator when compared to the traditional practice. The average cardiac cost of labor was decreased by 83.00 per cent with the utilization of groundnut decorticator. The work output was also found higher with the improved technology [24]. The study revealed that physiological stress output recorded by improved serrated sickle was average of 51.03 m^2/h as compared to local serrated sickle by which 37.52 m^2/h area was harvested. During harvesting with local sickle, the average ΔHR was 33.93 beats/min and energy expenditure was 12.33 kJ/s while by improved serrated sickle, it was recorded as 17.46 beats/min and 8.40 kJ/s. The average cardiac cost of work (CCW) was 55.41 beats/m^2 local sickle while 20.51 beats/m2 by improved serrated sickle. Therefore, the serrated sickle costs 35% less worker/unit of output and is 36.63% more efficient [25]. The study revealed that weeding through twin wheel hoe has proved efficient on time and output as compared with traditional Khurpi. The percentage change in average working heart rate was increased 18.88% with the use of twin wheel hoe. The output capacity was higher using twin wheel hoe (241.67 m^2/ hr) as compared to only (70.84 m^2/hr) with Khurpi; improved technologies have significantly higher work output than the traditional technology. It means that work output was near about thrice, as compared to traditional implement so working by twin wheel hoe is recommended. While performing weeding activity, average ΔHR was 10.00 beats/ min. While use of twin wheel hoe it was recorded as 27.00 beats/ min. The cardiac cost of worker was 8.00 beats/ m^2 while uses of twin wheel hoe it was 7.00 beats/ m^2. It is an accountable for energy expenditure during weeding in soybean crop and calculated energy expenditure was 7.27 kJ/min. Traditional practices, while by twin wheel hoe, it was recorded as 11.38 kJ/min and increases efficiency 247.45%.

4.2 Drudgery among rural women

Drudgery is usually conceived as physical and psychological strain, fatigue and monotony, hardship, experienced by humans. Drudgery of farm women is a crucial aspect that has attracted wide attention of researchers. If measured by the extensiveness and intensiveness of their involvement, farm women shoulder much more burden than man [26] does. Many of such activities are drudgery susceptible to varying degree. Even women suffer from different health problems, which adversely affect their working efficiency and family welfare. Women have shorter time to rest than men and environmental degradation is increasing women's work-load [27]. [28] also reported from Madhya Pradesh, India, participation of women in agriculture, India and developing countries are engaged in most of the farming and home related activities besides their exclusive involvement in domestic chores, women do the extremely tedious, time and labour intensive works. Generally, Indian women feel more work for a long time without rest and perform many roles in society and family. This drudgery or fatigue results in feeling tired, sleepiness, physical or mental stress, exhaustion and pain in body parts. So it are often said that each one the farm women suffer from the drudgery while performing various activities. [29] reported that women working in agriculture usually have to make do with archaic tools or a lack of proper tools at all which can also be unsafe, hazardous and unhealthy.

4.3 Physiological and psycho-physiological stress

While the mean average of heart rate when resting stationary remained at around 77–81 bpm, while working in the kitchen it ranged around 84–110 bpm while sitting down and 101–130 bpm while working standing up. In the kitchen, grinding turned out to be the most fatiguing work while vegetable-cutting was the friendliest for bpm [19]. Physiological stress on women while harvesting wheat activity averaged their heart rate to be around 121.5 b/min., which increased further up to 126.7 b/min. by the evening. Energy spent was also found to be 15.5 kJ/min, which further increased up to 12.3 kJ/min during evening hours [30]. It can be safely concluded that factors like bad state of workplace and lacking access to better tools contribute towards discomfort in both healthy and unhealthy individuals. These factors also greatly impact body posture, which alters the psychological functions of a private and produces many sorts of musculoskeletal problems. Agriculture work is expected to cause muscular-skeletal problems in developing countries [31].

4.4 Postural stress and Muscular-skeletal disorders in farm women

Muscular-skeletal disorder is observed to cause occupational ill-health as a leading factor. A bad posture is often cited as a factor causing the disorder in workplaces with prominent physical labour. The cervical spine, head and shoulders, elbow and wrist joint are all the parts, which can be related in the problems of efficiency, design, and discomfort. Muscular-skeletal issues are defined as damages to one's muscles, joints, tendons, or nerves, which can be an outcome of the many physical work-related factors. Early symptoms are pain, swelling, numbness, tingling, and loss of strength and range of motion. If one does not swift, the posture to the correct one it can cause acute and chronic issues. Acute problems are severe pain, excessive circulatory stress, and fatigue which could lead to higher chances of accidents and decreased productivity. Agriculture is generally recognized as the nation's most hazardous industry that displays high rates of musculoskeletal disorders with evidence to suggest that ergonomic risk factors are involved [32]. Chronic effects may produce many injuries and disorders in the musculoskeletal units, which may result in permanent or partial disability of the affected parts depending on the degree of stress and its duration [33]. The percentage deviation in the cervical region comes to1.7percentage to 7.3% among women belonging to 21–30 years. and 31–40 years of age groups while drawing water. In the lumber region the deviation was to the extent of 10and 8.9% leading to several musculoskeletal problems both in cervical and lumbar region [34]. [30] Stated that during the harvesting of wheat, women have to work in squatting posture from morning until evening. As they harvest wheat in this inconvenient position for long duration, there are high incidences of severe low back pain and pain in knees reported by these women [35]. Found that these issues were most frequently perceived in moderate to severe capacity as pain in shoulders, upper back, arms, and lower back while performing the work of threshing. Body Part Discomfort Score (BPDS) of both men and women in agriculture revealed that it was felt most severely in weeding, then in land preparation, followed by threshing, harvesting, irrigation and use of chemicals. On average, the Overall Discomfort Rating scores indicated that all the activities were in the range of 'high discomfort' both for men and women except irrigation where it was within the range of 'moderate discomfort' and therefore the ODR of females just in case of plant protection activity was within the range of 'light discomfort' [36]. Reported Indian farm women using of improved twin-wheel hoe for weeding in soybean crop reduce drudgery with muscular stress and fatigue. The focus of the demonstration was to vary the attitude, skill and knowledge towards recommended practices within the work. Farmwomen adopted the improved technique as it had increased the efficiency to work, reduce the drudgery and helped in avoiding bending or squatting posture. It lessened the exertion and fatigue to make the farmwomen conformable. [37] also revealed that massive number of workers suffered from low back trouble (93.3%), neck trouble (86.6%), wrist trouble (80%) and shoulder trouble (75%) due to the strenuous postures adopted while performing post harvesting jobs. [38] revealed that majority (33%) of the respondents performed the activities of planting/sowing, hand weeding, cutting/plucking, sorting and cleaning in bending, sitting or squatting postures. Mean many intensity of pain felt by respondents in several body parts different body parts revealed that respondents felt very mild (score-1) to very severe pain (score-5) in various body parts thanks to working in awkward postures for long durations. Hand weeding and cleaning of vegetables were rated as very demanding (mean score- 4.6); and planting/sowing, hand weeding and cleaning activities were very exhausting (mean score- 4.7, 4.6 and 4.8 respectively). Respondents adopted very difficult posture while planting/sowing; hand weeding, cutting/plucking and cleaning (mean score- 4.7, 4.6, 4.7 and 4.8 respectively). Planting/sowing and cutting/plucking were very painful activities (mean score 4.6); cutting/plucking was perceived as very heavy activity (mean score 4.6).

[39] concluded that both proper standing and bent posture were used by most farm-women while carrying out various activities like cutting (89%), threshing (37%) storage (45%), and Sun drying of grains (56%) respectively. While sowing (57%) and preparing land for threshing (74%), both squatting and bending posture had to be used while only bending posture was used or uprooting of seedlings (95%) and transplanting (96%). Most women used sitting posture for winnowing (92%), sieving (95%) and cleaning (96%). According to [40], women experienced severe to very severe pain in shoulder, upper arm, low back wrist/hands and knees while topdressing fertilizers using the traditional method instead of improved modern ones. The girls using modern methods to when fertilizing the farms showed a significant decline in experiencing pain (91.42%). Therefore most women experience moderate severe to severe pain in neck, shoulder, lower back, upper leg, calf muscles, wrist and ankle while working in agriculture.

4.5 Improved techniques and technologies on drudgery of women

Women in agriculture point to the fact that women are generally employed in the operations, which are either not mechanized or least mechanized and involve a lot of drudgery [41]. According to [42] the average physical cost of labour was less using the chaff cutter, sickle, Bhindi Plucker, seed treatment drum, weeder and groundnut stripper. Using Shovel, paddy thresher and wheelbarrow technologies, there was observed an increase in labour cost compared to old techniques. Work output saw rose with these modern methods except in the case of chaff cutter and seed treatment drum. Women generally had a positive response to using these methods as well. [18] reported use of groundnut decorticator reduced drudgery 84.26 per cent and it also saves time by 96.00 per cent in comparison to traditional practice. [43] study on drudgery reducing farm implements operated by women liked improved sickle and tubular maize cob sheller were carried results revealed that, 75% perceived the sickle as profitable (78.33%), compatible (76.77%), triable (75%) and observable (73.33%). Regarding the utilization of tubular maize cob sheller, 61.67% perceived the unit as profitable, compatible (73.33%), neither simple nor complex (58.33%), triable (66.67%) and observable (58.33%). Both sickle and tubular maize cob sheller were most feasible by majority of the farm women. Improved farm equipment that are women friendly are better in every respect in harvesting the crop. [44] Reported use of Naveen sickle, is best than the local sickle. It cover more area in given time, minimizes the drudgery and therefore the perceived exertion was low. It saves time and money expenditure on labour. It is very easy to handle and body problems are less.

As per [45], women participated most heavily in works such as seed treatment, transplantation, raising nursery, weeding, pruning, grain storage, manual harvesting, picking of vegetables, collection of animal dung and its transportation to fields. The knowledge level of participants about drudgery reducing implements was almost nil. After being trained, the women showed a 74.6% increase in level of knowledge about drudgery reduction. Saving time thus also lead them to make time to resting and take care of households. [46] reported hexagonal tubular maize Sheller saves almost half the time and increases working efficiency 30.25 per cent and reduces 70.60 per cent drudgery of farm women over traditional practice. It is also seen that maize sheller saves time by 23.78% as compared to traditional practice. [47] another study on hexagonal tubular maize sheller increased working efficiency 79.24 per cent and reduces 87.94 per cent drudgery of farm women over traditional practice. The cleaning efficiency was also increased 6.6% while using hexagonal tubular maize sheller. [25] revealed that drudgery was reduced 70. 21% when twin wheel hoe is used in weeding, it also reduce physiological cost, 21.42%, saves time 71.20% compared to traditional practice (Khurpi) while weeding in soybean crop.

4.6 Perception of Workload of agriculture activities

Physiological cost of operation is influenced by the health of operators, nutrition, basal rate and energy expended while working which will be indirectly measured by measuring oxygen consumption and pulse. Generally, person's subjective experience of a specific workload or rate of labor is more closely associated with pulse than to oxygen consumption during the performance of labor. Therefore, several research workers [48–52] have used pulse for assessment of physiological workload of the workers. [22] Indicated that farm women perceived significantly lowered exertion while performing the chosen farm activities with the improved tools compared to the utilization of traditional tools. According to this study [53], the impact of drudgery on women is that many respondents suffer from heavy physical strain and physical stress due to work overload i.e. 88.34 percent and 98.34 percent in Tarai and hill area. In addition, fewer respondents have the problem related with incidence of miscarriage i.e. 10 and 12 percent in Tarai and hill.

4.7 Perceived health hazards problems faced by farm workers

Occupational hazard constitutes a serious source of morbidity and mortality among all workers [54]. The occupational hazard could also be mainly thanks to two reasons i.e. the utilization of harmful chemicals in farming and biomechanical and posture demand of their health [55]. [56] also observed that farm women worked constantly in awkward postures during different agricultural activities then they suffered from discomfort in various parts of their body. [57] reported for occupational hazard among farm women were majority 65.00 per cent reported injury while harvesting followed by 33.33 per cent while weeding and 25.00 per cent while cleaning land. Joint problem was reported by 89.16 per cent farm women in wrist, 88.33 per cent in knee, back bone and shoulder, 75.00 per cent in neck and 73.33 per cent in elbow. Majority of farm women reported physical problems like body pain (95.83 per cent), tiredness (92.50 per cent) and physical stress (90.83 per cent) while transplanting. Farm women also reported impact of disease of the skin during farm activities i.e. heat stroke (84.16 per cent), heat prostration (68.33 per cent) and mycosis and allergy (23.33 per cent). [46] reported hexagonal tubular maize sheller shows easy in operation no muscle strain, low cardiac cost, less energy expenditure while using traditional practice. [25] revealed that Twin wheel hoe was user friendly tool can help to reduce the environmental an occupational health hazards of farm activity and also improved the work efficiency of workers during agriculture activities.

5. Conclusions

In this chapter, we shed light on farm women engaged in more time on post-harvest activities than those pre-harvest activities. Environmental and occupational health issues among agricultural workers expressed high levels of concern about working in warm weather, agricultural injuries, pesticides, awkward posture and drudgery prone activities. Improved drudgery agriculture tools saves time and money spend on labour, minimizes body muscular problems and it is very easy to handle. The probabilities of the injury are eliminated and it is safe to use thanks to its better construction and low cost effecting harvesting tool. This advanced technology might be adopted by the farm women. We still have an extended thanks to make a secure agricultural environment more efforts are needed for getting to availability of eco-friendly tools to finish users and thus, more emphasis on focusing ergonomists, agriculture experts, tool designers and organizations concerned with occupational health hazards.

Conflict of interest

The authors declare no conflict of interest.

Author statement

All authors read, reviewed, agree and approved the final manuscript.

Author details

Surendra Prasad Tripathi[1*†], Surya Pratap Singh Somvanshi[2†], Shyam Ranjan Kumar Singh[3†] and Anupam Mishra[4†]

1 KVK - Mandsaur, RVS Agriculture University, Gwalior, Madhya Pradesh, India

2 KVK - Hamirpur, Banda University of Agriculture and Technology University, Banda, Uttar Pradesh, India

3 ICAR, ATARI, Zone-IX, Jabalpur, Madhya Pradesh, India

4 Central Agricultural University, Imphal, Manipur, India

*Address all correspondence to: surya.somvanshi@gmail.com

† All authors equally contributed.

References

[1] Census report. Available at Registrar general of India, census, 2001, government of India 2011. Available at http://censusindia.gov.in/Census_And_You/economic_activity.aspx. 2017

[2] Prakash N, Singh R, Punitha KP, Roy SS, Ansari MA, Ngachan SV. Gender mainstreaming in small farm production system. Souvenir: 7th National Extension Education Congress in Umiam, Meghalaya. 2014

[3] Singh D, Vinay D, Gender Participation in Indian agriculture: An ergonomic evaluation of occupational hazard of farm and allied activities. International Journal of Agriculture, Environment and Biotechnology. 2013; **6**: 157

[4] Munshi, Sugandha. It's time to recognize and empower Indian's women farmers. World Economic Forum. 2017; **1**: 10 https://www.weforum.org/agenda/2017/10/indias-women-farmers

[5] Gautam US, Khare N, Singh A, Deva K. Technological module for farm women of Madhya Pradesh.Published by Directorate of Extension Services, JNKVV, and Jabalpur. 2008; 222 p

[6] IEA, International Ergonomics Association: Triennial report, Santa Monica, CA: IEA Press. 2000

[7] Mrunalini A, Choudhary S. Drudgery experiences of gender in crop production activities Journal of Agriculture Sciences. 2010; **1**: 49-51.

[8] Singh S. P. Drudgery alleviating: Farm tools and implements. Indian Farm 2012; **61**: 19-20

[9] Chaudhary RC, Srivastava AK, Yadav SK, Mishra SB. International Journal of Agriculture Science, 2018; **10**: 5390 – 5392.

[10] Garrow J. Human nutrition and dietetics. Nutrition News 1991. National Institute of Nutrition, Hyderabad. 1987

[11] [11]Snedecor, G. Cochran, W. Cox, D. 1989. Statistical Methods (8th edition). The Iowa State University Press

[12] Singh SP, Gite LP, Majumder J, Agarwal N. Aerobic capacity of Indian farm women using sub-maximal exercise technique on tread mill. Agricultural Engineering International: The CIGR E-Journal, X. 2008.

[13] Saha PN The practical use of some physiological research methods for assessment work stress. Journal of Indian Association of Physiotherapists. 1976; **4**: 9-13

[14] Corlett EN, Bishop RP. A technique for assessing postural discomfort. Ergonomics. 1976; **19**: 175-182.

[15] Nataraju MS, Lovely, PG. Role of farm women in farm and household activities. Interaction.1989; **50**: 19-20.

[16] Manekar K. Women and employment. Employment News, 1990; **6**: 7-13

[17] [17]Badiger C, Huilgol S. Nature and extent of women's involvement in agriculture and animal husbandry activities. Indian research Journal of Extension Education. 2004; **4**:124-128

[18] Tripathi SP, Tiwari J, Tripathi S, Somvanshi SPS. Drudgery reduction of farm women through groundnut decorticator. Research in Environment and Life Science. 2016c; **9:** 1501-1503

[19] Varghese MA, Chatterjee L, Atreya N, Bhatnagar A. Anthropometry and its ergonomic implications, DRS project report, Department of Family

Resource Management, SNDT Women's University, Bombay. 1989

[20] Murali D, Boki VI Kulkarni MS. Physiologicalcost of selected household and farm activities by rural women. Journal of Maharashtra Agriculture 2007; **3**: 449-450

[21] Nag PK, Sebastian NC, Maulankar MG. Occupational workload of Indian agriculture workers. Ergonomics.1980; **23**:91-102.

[22] Hasalkar S, Budihal R, Shivalli R, Biradar N. Assessment of work load of weeding activity in crop production through heart rate. Journal of Human Ecology. 2004; **14**: 165-167

[23] Chauhan MK, Workload and health problems in some occupational activities. Paper presented in Advanced Training Course in Ergonomics, at SNDT Women's University, Mumbai. 1999

[24] Tripathi SP, Somvanshi SPS, Mishra Anupam, Singh SRK Verma S. Ergonomic Evaluation of Farm Women through Improved Serrated Sickle for Harvesting in Wheat. Journal of Community Mobilization and Sustainable Development. 2015b; **10**: 233-236

[25] Tripathi SP, Chundawat GS, Somvanshi SPS, Shrivastava DC. Drudgery reduction of farm women through twin wheel hoe for weeding in soybean crop Research in Environment and Life Science. 2016a; **9**: 819-821

[26] Chandra N, Joshi P, Jethi R, Roy ML, Kharbikar HL, Atheequlla GA. Health and Nutritional Issues of Hill Farm Women: A Socio Economic Paradigm. International Journal of Agriculture and Food Science Technology. 2013; **4**: 431 – 438

[27] Mariama A, Janet H. Gender and the environment: Women's time use as a measure of environment change, Global environmentchange 1995; **5**: 337 – 346

[28] Mishra A, Singh, SRK Singh, Borker AJ Gour S. Inventory on women friendly tools. ICAR- ATARI, Jabalpur. 2016; 40

[29] Nag PK, Nag A. Drudgery, accidents and injuries in Indian agriculture. Industrial Health. 2004; **42**:149-162.

[30] Jyotsna KR, Singh K, Mehta M. Ergonomic Evaluation of the Rural Women While Performing Wheat Harvesting Activity Journal of Human Ecology. 2005; **18**: 309-311

[31] Suthar N, Kaushik V. Musculo skeletal problems among agricultural female workers Studies Home &Community Science. 2013;**7**: 145-149.

[32] Kishtwaria J, Rana A. Cutting and uprooting tasks of hill women: Stresses and solutions. In: Developments in agricultural and industrial ergonomics Women at work, edited by Gite LP, Mehta CR, Kotwaliwale N and Majumder J. (Allied publishers Pvt ltd.), 2007; **2**: 34-42

[33] Varghese MA, Atreya N, Saha PN. An Ergonomic evaluation of workload on selected meal preparation at two different heights of kitchen preparation at two different heights of platform, Dept. of FRM. SNDTWomen's University, Mumbai. 1996.

[34] AICRP Ergonomics of farm women's drudgery. Annual Report Deptof F.R.M., CCS HAU, Hisar.Haryana. 1999.

[35] Vyas R. Ergonomic Assessment of Prevalence of Musculoskeletal Disorders among Indian Agricultural Workers. Journal of Ergonomics Sciences.2014; **4**: 2165-7556.

[36] Sharma B, Singh SRK, Gupta S, Shrivastava MK, Verma S. Improving efficiency and reduction in drudgery of farm wom en in weeding activity by

twin wheel Hoe. Indian research Journal of Extension. 2015; **15**: 76-80

[37] Maiti D, Sau S, Dhara PC. Musculoskeletal Disorders and Postural Stress in Post Harvesting Jobs. In: Proceedings of Humanizing Work and Work Environment, HWWE, (CIAE, Bhopal) Edited by Gite L P, Mehta CR, Kotwaliwale N and Majumder J. 2007, 89-95

[38] Gupta R, Bisht D. Postural stress and work-related musculoskeletal disorders of female labors working in agricultural fields with traditional methods The Pharma Innovation Journal 2018; **7:** 252-255

[39] Borah R, and kalita, M. Identifying Drudgery Prone Home Activities in Rural Areas of Upper Brahmaputra Valley Zone of Assam. Studies on Home Community Science. 2011. **5**: 165-168

[40] Hasalkar S, Rajeshwari S, Budihal R Musculo-Skeletal Disorders of the Farm Women While Performing the Top Dressing of Fertilizer Activity, Journal of Human Ecology. 2007; **21**: 109-112 DOI: 10.1080/09709274..11905958

[41] Singh SP, Gite LP. Ergonomical assessment of hand operated paddy winnower by woman workers. Journal of Agricultural Engineering (ISAE) 2007; **44**: 67-71.

[42] Badiger C, Hasalkar S, Huilgol S, Hoskeri M, Kavita P. Ergonomic assessment of improved agricultural technologies introduced for farm women in northern Karnataka. Published in the proceedings of international conference on emerging technologies in agricultural and food engineering, IIT. 2004

[43] Sharma Neetu Perception of farm women about feasibility of drudgery reducing farm implements. Annals of biology.2002; **18**: 209-210.

[44] Sharma B, Verma S, Mustafa Md. Ergonomic Evaluation of Drudgery Load Faced by Farm Women in Wheat Harvesting. International Journal of Current Microbiology Applied Science. 2017; 6: 3014-3022. doi: https://doi.org/10.20546/ijcmas.2017.610.355

[45] Kumar S, Srivastava AK, Mishra SB, Chaudhary RC. Reducing Drudgery of Farmwomen through Appropriate Farm Implements in Uttar Pradesh, India. International Journal of Agriculture Sciences. 2018; **10:** 5761-5764

[46] Tripathi SP, Somvanshi SPS, Gupta S, Verma S. Ergonomics study through tubular maize sheller of farm women in Mandsaur (M.P.). Progressive Research – An International Journal 2015a;**10**: 3099-3101

[47] Tripathi SP, Somvanshi SPS, Bhadhoria UPS, Singh A. Ergonomic Evaluation of Hand Operated Maize Sheller On Farm Women Of Mandsaur District (M.P.). Plant Archives 2016b; **16**: 303-305

[48] Kathirvel K, Ananthakrishnan, D. Physiological cost of rice farming operations. All India Coordinated Research Project on Human Engineering and Safety In Agriculture. Progress Report 2000; **1**: 97-105

[49] Singh SP, Gite LP, Agarwal N. Ergonomical evaluation of manually-operated fertilizer broadcaster with farm women.Journal of Agricultural Engineering (ISAE). 2004; **41**: 22-25

[50] Singh SP, Gite LP, Agarwal N. Physiological Workload of Farm Women in the Operation of CIAE Hanging Type Cleaner. Book Chapter entitled "Power Machinery Systems and Ergonomics, Safety and Health" Amanya Publication, New Delhi, 2005; pp 343-347.

[51] Singh SP, Gite LP, Agarwal N. Ergonomical assessment of manually operated seed drills for farm women.

Journal of Agricultural Engineering (ISAE). 2006; **43:** 42-48.

[52] Singh SP, Gite LP, Agarwal N, Majumder J. Women friendly improved farm tools and equipment Technical bulletin no. Published by CIAE, Bhopal India. 2007; **128**: 56 p.

[53] Pant K, Kwatra J, Kwatra S. Occupational health hazards of hill women of Uttarakhand engaged in farm activities. The Pharma Innovation Journal 2020; **9**: 08-10

[54] Driscoll T, J Takala, K Steenland, CorvalanC, Fingerhut M. Review of estimates of global burden of injury and illness due to occupational exposures. American Journal of Industrial Medicine. 2005; **48**: 491-502

[55] Menon S, Sheshadri. Report of National Task force on Technological empowerment of women in Agriculture. 2004

[56] Nidhi, Kaushik V. Ergonomic study on postures used by farm women in vegetable cultivation. Abstract 14th International Conference on Humanizing Work and Work Environment HWWE, 2016; **11**: 67-68.

[57] Singh P, Dubey SK, Pandey S. Occupational Health Hazard among Farm Women in Kannauj district of Uttar Pradesh. Journal of Community Mobilization and Sustainable Development 2019; **14**: 5-10

Chapter 5

Ergonomic Evaluation of Thermal Stress in a Tunisian Steel Industry

Amira Omrane, Taoufik Khalfallah and Lamia Bouzgarrou

Abstract

This work aims to assess thermal stress based on the various measurable thermal stress parameters (wet bulb temperature, air speed, radiation temperature, black globe temperature...). A cross-sectional study was carried in a steel company. The evaluation of thermal stress was made by physical parameters measurment (air temperature, relative humidity, air velocity, globe temperature, clothing insulation, metabolism of work) and analyzed according to the International Standard Organization (ISO) 7933 "Analytical determination and interpretation of heat stress using calculation of the predicted heat strain". Eighty male workers were mean ageed of 37.9 ± 9.25 years. The climatic conditions category was three (meaning a Long-term stress) in 68.18% of the workers and four (Short-term stress meaning the occurrence of health problems within 30 to 120 minutes of exposure) in 30.3% of workers. The long and short-term thermal stress identified in this study spearhead a prevention strategy (automation of manufacturing processes, improvement of the organization of tasks, and the strengthening of medical surveillance of workers).

Keywords: ergonomics, thermal stress, steel industry, international standard organisation, prevention

1. Introduction

Historically, the arduous sectors of work described have been physically heavy such as work in the steel industry. In this context, this arduousness is related to significant thermal constraints caused by the production processes. In Tunisia, this sector employs more than 2498 workers [1]. Currently, the available tools for quantifying strain and thermal stresses are the result of a great research at the origin of European directive 89/654/EEC and of 14 standards developed by the International Standard Organization (ISO) [1–3]. This large number of thermal stress assessment tools reflect the complexity of prediction models and the difficulties in defining a simple model that can be used in various work situations [2]. This work was encouraged by the importance of the thermal constraints in the steel sector, the characteristics of the climate in Tunisia especially in the hot season and the employability of this sector. This research was conducted in the governorate of Monastir. It has a dry mediterranean climate with hot summers, extremely mild winters, much sunshine and low rainfall year-round. The city sits in the northeast of Tunisia, on its central coast. The average high temperature of 29°C (84°F) in June skips past the 30°C (86°F) mark in the middle of the month and rises to 33°C (91°F) in July and August.

This work aims to assess thermal stress based on the various measurable thermal stress parameters (wet bulb temperature, air speed, radiation temperature, black globe temperature...).

2. Materials and methods

This is an exhaustive cross-sectional study carried out during the two months of August and September 2015, in a Tunisian steel company specialized in the manufacture of springs for heavy vehicles and located in the industrial zone of Teboulba-Moknine of the governorate of Monastir, Tunisia. This company counted 120 workers. A list of names and contact details of all workers was provided by the Human Resources Management Department. Included patients were those who had a job tenure exceeding one year and belonged to production workshops. Exclusion criteria consisted of a participation refusal and a disability or cognitive impairment precluding participation.

The survey was preceded by an individual interview with each eligible worker in order to explain the objectives of the work, its practical progress, guarantee anonymity and obtain informed consent. During the survey, data collection focused on general characteristics, as well as thermal stress measurements. Data analysis was subsequently carried out by the same investigator, using statistical and computer programs.

2.1 Data collection

1. General characteristics related to age, weight, height, Body Mass Index (BMI)...

2. Measurement of the thermal environment carried out in the workstation of each worker and in the external environment (rest area during recovery breaks). These recordings were preceded by open observation days to estimate the actual duration of the activity set at five hours. Open observation also enabled a contact with the operators and the collection of their opinions concerning the time and extent of the temperature peak. The thermal stress mainly concerns the morning and afternoon shiftwork and extended from 7 am to 7 pm. Thus, measurements were made every 15 minutes at the workstations. The values obtained were means of all measurements performed. These measurements were carried out in accordance with the ISO 7726 standard "*Ergonomics of the thermal environment - Instruments for measuring physical quantities*" [4] using:

    - a thermo-hygrometer (TA5 Thermal Anemometers) placed at the workstation at a height of 1.5 m, far from the employees and sheltering the sensor against radiation (sun, oven, etc.). It is a calibrated device with a low response time, a stabilization time of a few seconds enabling punctual measurement of air temperature and relative humidity.

    - a vane anemometer (YK-80AP Vane Anemometer) for measuring air speed. The measurement was discontinuous and the axis of rotation was placed in the direction of the air flow.

- a black globe thermometer (Black globe TP_875.1/TP_876.1) placed at the work station at a height of 1.5 m, keeping the employees apart. The measurement time is about 20 min.

2.2 Thermal stress analysis

This evaluation was conducted by the program "Ergonomics of work in heat - Calculation of PMV indices - PPD, WBGT and P.H.S." developed by Prof. Malchaire [5] and based on the various physical parameters of the thermal environment (air temperature, black globe temperature, relative humidity, speed of air) as well as on:

- The equivalent metabolism M estimated based on the ISO 8996 standard "Ergonomics of the thermal environment - Determination of energy metabolism" [6].

- Iclo clothing insulation assessed in accordance with the ISO 9920 standard "Ergonomics of the thermal environment - Determination of thermal insulation and resistance to evaporation of a clothing" [7] Thus, the program identifies the parameters:

    - Predicted Mean Vote (PMV) at work and during recovery. This PMV index predicts the average vote value of a large group of people on the following seven-point thermal sensation scale: + 3 very hot; + 2 hot; + 1 slightly hot; 0 neither hot nor cold; −1 slightly cold; −2 cold; −3 very cold [1]

    - Predicted Percentage of Dissatisfied (PPD) in the workplace and during recovery. This PPD index is defined as the percentage of people who, placed in identical conditions, consider themselves cold/very cold or hot/very hot. These are the people who would have cast a vote outside the interval (−1, 1) on the sensation scale [1]. To obtain a thermal comfort situation, it is recommended that the PPD be less than 10%, which corresponds to a PMV between −0.5 and + 0.5 [1].

    - Thermal sensation in work situation and during recovery: This index is calculated from the PMV and PPD indices and In accordance with ISO 7730 "Ergonomics of the thermal environments - Analytical determination and interpretation of thermal comfort by calculating the PMV and PPD indices and by local thermal comfort criteria" [8].

    - The natural humid temperature (Thn) in work situation and during recovery.

    - The Wet Bulb Globe Temperature (WBGT) in the workplace and during recovery. The WBGT corresponds to a weighting between the radiation temperature and the natural wet bulb temperature.

$$\begin{aligned} \text{WBGT} &= 0.7\ \text{thn} + 0.3\ \text{tg without solar R} \\ &= 0.7\ \text{thn} + 0.2\ \text{tg} + 0.1\ \text{ta with solar R} \end{aligned} \quad (1)$$

    - The WBGT limits in work situation and during recovery

The working hours - rest limits (K): This duration is calculated in accordance with ISO 7243 "Hot environments - Estimation of the thermal stress of man at work, based on the WBGT index (wet bulb and black globe temperature)" [9] and according to the following equation:

$$K = \frac{32 - WBGT}{32 - WBGT_{lim}} \quad (2)$$

- o Sweat flow in a work situation and during recovery.
- o Total water loss in the workplace and during recovery
- o The time interval indicated for drinking 200 cc of water at 10°C
- o The core temperature reached after 8 hours of work
- o The time interval to achieve excessive water loss
- o The time interval to reach a core temperature of 38°C.
- o The climatic condition categories in the work situation and during recovery: Identified in five levels in accordance with ISO 7933 "Analytical determination and interpretation of heat stress using calculation of the predicted heat strain" [10]:

    a. C1: Comfort category: neither discomfort nor health risk;

    b. C2: Discomfort category: discomfort that can be very significant, but without health risk;

    c. C3: Category of long-term constraint: discomfort and risk of dehydration after several hours of exposure;

    d. C4: Short-term stress category: health risk after 30 to 120 minutes of exposure;

    e. C5: Immediate Constraint Category: health risk even for very short exposure (less than 30 minutes)

3. Results

3.1 Study population

The survey was carried out exhaustively among the operators of the production workshops of the steel company, and included a total of 80 male workers. The mean age was 37.9 ± 9.25 years and the mean professional tenure was 12.5 ± 11.4 years (**Table 1**).

3.2 Evaluation of thermal stress

This stress was evaluated based on the different physical parameters of the thermal environment (air temperature, temperature of the black globe, relative

Characteristics	
Men	80
Mean age ± (extremes)	37,9 ± 9,25 years (from 21 to 54 years)
Groups: n(%) • **Men > 45 years:** • **Men < 45 years:**	62 (77,5%) 18 (12,5%)
Married Depending children: • 0 **child** • 1 **to** 3 **children** • ≥3 **children**	61 (76,25%) 10 (12,5%) 27 (33,75%) 24 (30%)
Mean job tenure ± (extremes)	12,5 ± 11,4 years (from1 to 35 years).
Mean BMI ± (extremes) • **Normal** • **Overweight** • **Obesity**	26,9 ± 3,6 kg/m^2 (17,8 à 38,7 kg/m2) 19 (23.75%) 49 (61,25%) 12(15%).

Table 1.
Study population.

humidity, and air speed) as well as on the equivalent metabolism M and the Iclo clothing insulation index evaluated in accordance with the ISO 9920 standard "Ergonomics of the thermal environment - Determination of thermal insulation and resistance to evaporation of a clothing" [7].

1. *Thermal environment*: The mean air temperature inside the workshops was 29.66 ± 2.57°C with a mean air speed of 0.58 ± 0.82 m/s, a mean relative humidity of 59, 56 ± 10.98 and a mean global temperature of 34.15 ± 2.87°C (**Table 2**).

2. *Thermal stress evalation*: Based on the evaluation of the equivalent metabolism and the characteristics of the thermal environment, the thermal stress to which the workers of the different production workshops were exposed, was evaluated by the indices of Predicted Mean Vote (PMV) and Predicted Percentage of Dissatisfied (PPD) as follows (**Table 3**):

    - Mean PMV of 3.2 ± 0.47 with extremes ranging from 1.5 to 4.7.

    - Mean PPD 97.3 ± 3.7% with extremes of 50 to 100%.

    Thereby:

    - The Thermal sensation was rated "very hot" on 98.75% of all working days.

    - The mean WBGT was 27.5 ± 2.62°C

    - The mean WBGT limit 28.4 ± 0.81°C. Based on previous estimates, and in accordance with ISO 7243 "Hot environments - Estimation of the thermal stress of humans at work, based on the WBGT index (wet bulb and black globe temperature)" [9], the mean cut-off working time was evaluated at 48 ± 13.19 min.

	In door	Out door
Mean air temperature (Ta) (°C)	29,66 ± 2,57	27,99 ± 1,87
Mean air speed (Va) (m/s)	0,58 ± 0,82	0,23 ± 0,26
Mean relative humidity (RH) (%)	59,56 ± 10,98	68, 56 ± 7,78
Mean Globe temperature (Tg) (°C)	34, 15 ± 2,87	40,21 ± 7,95

Table 2.
Physical parameters of thermal stress.

	Minimum	Maximum	Mean	Standard deviation
PMV	1,5	4,7	3,2	0,47
PPD (%)	50	100	97,3	3,7
WBGT (°C)	20	29,9	27,5	2,62
Limit WBGT (°C)	26,5	30,2	28,4	0,81
Work limit time/60 min (min)	3	60	48	13,19
Sweat loss (g/h)	230	1130	699,4	160,03
Total water loss (g)	1780	10600	6083,7	1737,3
Time interval Indicated to drink 200 cc of water at 10 °C (min)	10	55	19,4	5,49
Central temperature after 8 hours of work (°C)	37,3	42	38,6	1,03
Time to reach excessive water loss (min)	160	480	292,6	74,64
The central temperature reaches 38°C at the end of (min)	46	385	131,3	60,89

Table 3.
Thermal stress evaluation.

In addition, the mean sweat flow was 699.4 ± 160.02 g/h and the mean total water loss was estimated to be 6083.7 ± 1737.29 g.

In accordance with the recommendations of ISO 7933 "Analytical determination and interpretation of thermal stress based on the calculation of the foreseeable thermal strain", it would be imperative to offer all workers oral rehydration by water at 10°C after a calculated average working time of 19.4 ± 5.49 min.

According to these estimates, after 8 hours of work, the average core temperature would reach 38.6 ± 1.03°C. Excessive water loss was reported among 80.3% of workers and would be reached after 292.6 ± 74.64 min. The core temperature would be 38°C, based on these evaluations, among 51.5% of workers who received a heart rate recording after 131.3 ± 60.89 min.

In total, on the basis of these results of the estimation of thermal stresses, 68.18% of subjects would be concerned by a category 3 of climatic condition, namely "Long-term stress: discomfort and risk of dehydration after several hours of exposure" and 30. 3% of them by a category 4 of climatic condition equivalent to a "Short-term constraint: risk to health after 30 to 120 minutes of exposure".

4. Discussion

This study included measurements of the physical parameters of thermal stress followed by an evaluation of thermal stress. Informed consent from workers was obtained before the start of the study. The questionnaire survey enabled the identification of the main socio-demographic characteristics. In this study, thermal stress was evaluated by the PHS ISO 7933 index "Analytical determination and interpretation of heat stress using calculation of the predicted heat strain" [10]. The physical parameters used to calculate this index come from measurements of the environment as well as from the estimation of the equivalent metabolism in accordance with the ISO 8996 "Ergonomics of the thermal environment - Determination of energy metabolism".

The ISO 7933 standard provides a main advantage of the PHS model related to the reorganization of work, by interposing of short periods of rest during work and the distribution of drinks so as to compensate the water losses taking into account the interindividual differences in physiological responses to heat [1]. This model has been validated using data from 672 laboratory experiments and 237 field experiments [1, 11–13].

Thermal comfort is defined as a state of satisfaction against a person's thermal environment evaluated by six primary parameters providing this comfort [1]. This comfort was estimated by the PMV and PPD indices described by the ISO 7730 standard [8]. The results of this study were convincing, more than a half (65 operators) were not in a situation of thermal comfort.

It should be noted that the thermal stress is also estimated using the WBGT index described by the ISO 7243 standard [9]. This index has a fairly limited field of application, in particular while evaluating thermal stress during very short periods or conditions close to the thermal comfort [1]. The PHS model seems to be more discriminating than the WBGT index in defining the severity of thermal stress during work situation and organizing work in order to minimize or eliminate thermal stress. Metabolism value estimated for the calculation of this index comes from the results of the recording of the heart rate which gives it an accuracy of the order of ±10% and then an accurate estimation [14]. Therefore, only results of the PSH evaluation will be discussed in this work.

The climatic conditions category was 3 in 68.18% of subjects (Long-term constraint: discomfort and risk of dehydration after several hours of exposure) and 4 (Short-term constraint: health risk after 30 to 120 minutes of exposure) in 30.3% of workers. The use of this index enabled the assessment of the thermal stress and the management of work in heat [15]. Thus, workers were advised to drink water at 10° C after an average working time of 19.4 ± 5.49 min. A possible alternative is to let employees spontaneously choose their space of work or to allow them to stop working as soon as they feel some symptoms of strain [1, 16].

In this study population, the core temperature could reach 38°C after an average working time of 131.3 ± 60.89 min. The World Health Organization (WHO) Technical Report No. 412 published in 1969 stated that: "*It is not recommended that the core body temperature exceeds 38°C for prolonged daily exposure to heavy work…*" [4]. It should be emphasized that, at a rectal temperature of 38°C, an employee does not run any health risk. This limit value concerns the "average" subject and is intended to protect employees who, due to a greater intolerance to heat, evolve to higher temperatures, under the same conditions [1].

In this study, more than half of workers (58.75%) know nothing about the risks associated with working in the heat, while 10 employees have already had accidents due to heat (cramps, faintness, stroke. heat). Employees should be informed and trained to recognize signs of thermal stress and prevent the occurrence of these accidents [1, 17].

This study has limitations that warrant mentioning. The thermal stress evaluation was made by physical objective measurements that did not take into account operators' differences. Moreover, the investigation was limited to one company located in the central-eastern region of Tunisia. Therefore, findings cannot be extended to all of Tunisian companies, especially with the huge differences in weather, in characteristics and resources between sectors of activity, between industrial process and between operators.

5. Conclusion

In the light of our results and the literature data, several measures should be implemented in this steel company, to prevent both short-term and long-term effects linked to thermal stress in this environment.

Globally, the preventive approach in this sector must combine technical, organizational and medical actions. Its implementation must be multidisciplinary, involving, on the basis of the action plan proposed by the occupational physician, all of the experts involved in the development of work processes, the layout and design of workstations, such as production engineers, quality engineers, industrial hygienists, ergonomist, architects, but also the expert in the work situation; the operator himself.

Finally, additional study of thermal stress taking into account dependencies and synergistic factors and operators' differences should be performed.

Author details

Amira Omrane*, Taoufik Khalfallah and Lamia Bouzgarrou
Occupational Medicine and Ergonomics Department, Public Hospital Taher Sfar, Mahdia, Tunisia

*Address all correspondence to: amiraomrane20@gmail.com

References

[1] J. Malchaire, Work in the heat, EMC-Toxicologie Pathologie 1 (2004) 96–116

[2] C Martinet, JP Meyer. Travail à la chaleur et confort thermique. Note scientifiques et techniques 184 (1999). www.inrs.fr/dms/inrs/Publication/NOETUDE-3641-01/ns184.pdf consulted 25 february 2017

[3] Directive 89/654/CEE du Conseil, du 30 novembre 1989, concernant les prescriptions minimales de sécurité et de santé pour les lieux de travail (première directive particulière au sens de l'article 16 paragraphe 1 de la directive 89/391/CEE). Journal Officiel n L 393 du 30/12/1989. p. 0001-0012.

[4] Norme ISO 7726. Ergonomie des ambiances thermiques - Appareils de mesure des grandeurs physiques. 1998.

[5] Malchaire J. Occupational Heat Stress Assessment by the Predicted Heat Strain Model. Industrial Health 2006; 44: 380-387.

[6] International Standard Organization, ISO 8996, Determination of metabolic rate, Genève: ISO; 2004.

[7] International Standard Organization 9920. Ergonomics of the thermal environment — Estimation of thermal insulation and water vapour resistance of a clothing ensemble. 2007.

[8] International Standard Organization 7730. Ergonomics of the thermal environment — Analytical determination and interpretation of thermal comfort using calculation of the PMV and PPD indices and local thermal comfort criteria. 2005.

[9] International Standard Organization 7243. Ergonomics of the thermal environment — Assessment of heat stress using the WBGT (wet bulb globe temperature) index. 2017.

[10] International Standard Organization 7933. Ergonomics of the thermal environment — Analytical determination and interpretation of heat stress using calculation of the predicted heat strain. 2004.

[11] Malchaire J, Kampmann B, Mehnert P, Gebhardt H, Piette A, Havenith G, et al. Évaluation du risque de contrainte thermique lors du travail en ambiances chaudes. Méd Hyg Trav Ergon 2001;XXXVIII:101–112.

[12] Malchaire J, Piette A, Kampmann B, Mehnert P, Gebhardt H, Havenith G, et al. Development and validation of the predicted heat strain model. Ann Occup Hyg 2001;45:123–135.

[13] Malchaire J, Kampmann B, Mehnert P, Gebhardt H, Piette A, Havenith G, et al. Assessment of the risk of heat disorders encountered during work in hot conditions. Int Arch Occup Environ Health 2002;75:153–162.

[14] Jacques MALCHAIRE, Francesca Romana d'AMBROSIO ALFANO and Boris Igor PALELLA. Evaluation of the metabolic rate based on the recording of the heart rate. Ind Health. 2017; 55(3): 219–232. doi: 10.2486/indhealth.2016-0177

[15] Pongjan Yoopat, K. Vanwonterghem and K. Intaranont, An assessment of workload in the Thai steel industry, Applied Ergonomics, 1998: 29 (4) 267-271

[16] Mairiaux P, Malchaire J. Comparison and validation of heat stress indices in experimental studies. Ergonomics 1995;38:58–72.

[17] Kaija Tuomi, Sinikka Vanhala,Erkki Nykyri and Minna Janhonen. Organizational practices, work demands and the well-being of employees: a follow-up study in the metal industry and retail trade. Occup Med 2004; 54: 115-121.

Chapter 6

Responsiveness of Occupational Health Risk and Preventive Measures Practice by the Workers Employed in Tannery Occupation in Kanpur, India

Gyan Chandra Kashyap, Praveen Chokhandre and Shri Kant Singh

Abstract

Occupational health covers all aspects of health and safety in the workplace and has a strong focus on primary prevention of hazards. The objective of the study was to understand the extent of awareness about occupational health risks involved in tannery occupation and adopted preventive measures by the tannery workers of Kanpur, India. Information for the present research was strained from a cross-sectional household study of tannery workers in the Jajmau area of Kanpur. The survey was piloted through the period January–June 2015, and 284 samples were collected. The prevalence of awareness of tannery work is very hazardous in nature varies from 73–93% among the tannery workers. Tannery workers having a middle-school level of education were 3.01 times more likely to be aware of the hazards as compared to the illiterate workers. Tannery workers aged 36 and above were less likely to aware of a hazardous work environment. Further, tannery workers who belong to the younger cohort (16–24 years) reported a higher awareness of respiratory problems (38%), skin complaints (59%), and gastrointestinal issues (21%) than those aged 36 years and above. About one-third of Beam house workers (33%) and over a quarter (26%) of the wet finishing had moderate to high dermal contact with the chemicals. The study's outcomes give a clear indication of the effect of the workstation environment on the health status of workers and require the use of adequate measures to improve the facilities and thereby the health status of tannery workers.

Keywords: Occupational health risk, preventive measures, tannery workers, work environment, health hazard, qualitative measure

1. Introduction

The enormous burden of poor working conditions stated by several studies and with the latest estimates provided by the International Labour Organization (ILO) that somewhere 2.3 million working people around the world capitulate to work-related accidents or diseases every year; this links to over 6000 deaths every single day. Worldwide, there are around 340 million occupational accidents and 160 million fatalities of work-related illnesses annually [1]. While improved and harmless workplaces can avoid at least 1.2 million deaths every year, according to 2018 world health organization (WHO) study [2]. Many causalities can be prevented through addressing significant health dangers, which is directly associated with the workplace, and the exposures such as stress, long working hours and shift work, prolonged sitting at work, work-related climate-sensitive diseases, such as heat and cold stress, as well as workplace air pollution [3–6].

Occupational health covers all aspects of health and safety in the workplace and has a strong focus on primary prevention of hazards. Depending on workplace conditions, there are several health risks: cancers, injuries/accidents, musculoskeletal disorders, respiratory problems, mental health disorders, skin ailments, infectious diseases, etc. Employment conditions in both formal and informal sectors are also significant factors: working hours, salary, and policies that cover such aspects as maternity leave, and provisions for protecting and promoting employee health [2]. Occupational health is a grave concern in developing countries, but there have been few studies of health issues faced by tannery workers because of which the problems are largely unknown. Further, the workers' health issues have not received sufficient attention from employers. The place and work environment are crucial influences on the extent of health risks faced by tannery workers. According to WHO, occupational health problems accounted for about 1.5 percent of the total burden of disease regarding disability adjusted life years (DALYs), particularly in occupational health, which included work-related injuries, and exposure to risks such as carcinogens, airborne particulates, ergonomic stressors, and noise [7].

Tannery workers are susceptible to multiple chemical and physical hazards in their work. Direct exposure to hazardous materials significantly increases health risks. The workers are exposed to chromium during the tanning process, leather dust, and various chemical agents. There are also ergonomic stressors that increase susceptibility to numerous health issues. Workers involved in multiple operations like material transfer, wet finishing, dry finishing, etc. are particularly vulnerable to harm. The risks associated with the tanning work is included in the proposed research paper examines the health hazards of tannery work Kanpur (India), and the preventive actions that are taken.

As mentioned earlier, there have been a limited number of studies of perceived health risks and preventive measures among tannery workers in the developing world. This research work investigates the work experience, working hours, type of job contract, and the type of work the tannery employees are usually engaged in. At the same time, it also examines their awareness of the hazardous work environment, the effect of exposure to chemicals, dangerous tissues involved in the tanning process. It also studies their perceptions of the effects of exposure to chemicals and contact with them, airborne dust, and ergonomic stressor. The objective of the study was to understand the extent of awareness about occupational health risks and adopted preventive measures during working hours among male tannery workers of Kanpur, India.

2. Methods

Information for the present research was strained from a cross-sectional household study of tannery workers in the Jajmau area of Kanpur, India. The survey was piloted through the period January–June 2015 and was a portion of a Ph.D.

database. All total of 284 tannery workers from the study area were questioned. Rigorous pre-testing was completed with the tannery workers of the Jajmau area for testing the internal uniformity of schedule. Beforehand starting the interviews, we have clarified the tenacity of the survey and requested to contribute to the study by giving the proper information. After that, face-to-face discussions were piloted among those who agreed to participate in the study by using a structured pre-tested questionnaire on the tannery workers.

2.1 Sampling design

This study has adopted a three-stage sampling design. At the first stage, seven localities in the Jajmau area, namely Tadbagiya, Kailash Nagar, J.K. colony, Asharfabad, Motinagar, Chabeelepurwa, and Budhiyaghat, were selected based on a higher concentration of leather tannery worker's population in these areas as reported by various stakeholders in the city. In the second stage, three out of the seven localities, namely Budhiyaghat, Tadbagiya, and Asharfabad, were selected by probability proportional to size (PPS) sampling technique after arranging them in increasing order of estimated number of HHs of leather tannery workers. Subsequently, a comprehensive household listing and mapping were completed in each of the three localities, and all the household were classified into three groups-*households having at least one tannery worker, irrespective of having or not having any non-tannery worker*, *households having non-tannery worker (s)* and *households having no worker*. The first two groups of households constituted two independent sampling frame in each of the three selected localities. While the third group of households was excluded from the study. Once the updated and comprehensive sampling frames were developed in each of the three areas included in the study, a circular systematic random sampling was used for the selection of households at the third and the last stage. In case, if more than one worker were in a household, the target respondent was selected using KISH table. In each of the three selected areas, 100 households were selected for each of the two categories i.e., a tannery as well as non-tannery workers, using a circular systematic random sampling procedure. Thus, a total of 600 HHs were selected for the interview, and a total of 284 HHs having at least tannery workers, and 289 HHs of non-tannery workers (s) were interviewed successively. In the paper, we have tried to understand the level of awareness among the leather tannery workers. Bivariate analysis and logistic regression analysis were performed.

Qualitative measurement of environmental exposures have been classified as follows: Chemicals in the air (no exposure, low exposure, moderate exposure, high exposure, very high exposure) was based on qualitative rating of exposure assessment as [0] No exposure: no contact with agent, agent is used in workplace but is very unlikely to result in exposure to workers involved. [1] Low exposure: infrequent contact with agent at low concentrations, Agent is used in a closed/controlled system; there are no specific activities that enhance exposure; exposure takes place because of presence at the shop floor. [2] Moderate exposure: frequent contact with agent at low concentrations, Agent is used throughout the closed/controlled process and exposure mainly occurs by passive contact; infrequent contact is needed with the agent. [3] High exposure: Frequent contact with agent at high concentrations, Nature of the production process and associated manual activities makes regular contact necessary; agent causes exposure during manual activities and around particular sources such as presses, drums. [4] Very high exposure: Frequent contact with agent at very high concentrations, Agent is used in manual activities that introduce frequent peak exposures such as cleaning, opening a press, spraying paint.

2Dermal exposure to chemicals (no exposure, moderate exposure, high exposure) was based on qualitative rating of exposure assessment as [0] No skin contact: no contact with agent. [1] Moderate exposure: infrequent skin contact with agent contact occurs during specific activities that are not part of the daily work routine. [2] High exposure: frequent skin contact with agent regular contact is unavoidable due to particular activities in daily work practice. 3Another important variable airborne dust (no exposure, low exposure, moderate exposure, high exposure, very high exposure) was based on qualitative rating of exposure assessment as [0] No exposure: clear visibility. [1] Low exposure: visibility more than 10 m. [2] Moderate exposure: visibility between 5 to 10 m. [3] High exposure: visibility between 1 to 5 m. [4] Very high exposure: visibility less than 1 m. 4Ergonomic stressors (no exposure, low exposure, moderate exposure, high exposure, very high exposure) was based on qualitative rating of exposure assessment as [0] No exposure: does not occur (< 10% of work time). [1] Low exposure: less than 25% of daily work time. [2] Moderate exposure: 25–49% of daily work time. [3] High exposure: 50–74% of daily work time. [4] Very high exposure: 75% or more of daily work time. Exposure of waste water of chromium (no exposure, moderate exposure, high exposure) was based on qualitative rating of exposure assessment as [0] No exposure: no contact with chromium water. [1] Moderate exposure: infrequent contact with chromium water. [2] High exposure: frequent contact with chromium water.

2.2 Data analysis

We begin with the descriptive analysis (frequency distribution) to present the sample. Further, cross-tabulation was done to study the association with the dependent variable and predictor variables included in the study. Adjusted odds ratio from the binary logistic regression was executed to determine the associated factors. Data were analyzed using STATA 14 software.

3. Results

3.1 Work related characteristics of tannery workers

The work-related characteristics of tannery workers are presented in **Table 1**. Tannery operations was categorized into four broad categories: Beam house work (8% of workers in a tannery unit), wet finishing (25%), dry finishing (50%), and miscellaneous work (17%).

We collected information on total work experience (in the present job and previous ones) in tanneries. Around 15 percent of the tannery workers surveyed were engaged in the occupation for more than 20 years, and about one-third of workers were involved for 20 years in the tannery occupation. Most of the workers (89%) were working as daily wage laborers, while only 11 percent were permanent employees. Over one-fourth (27%) worked for 11 to 12 hours a day, and 52 percent reported that they worked for all seven days in the week.

The nature of the work done is shown in **Figure 1**. For this study, the job contract was divided into two categories—temporary (daily wages) and permanent. Most workers were engaged in works on a temporary basis. In the beam house, where the work is particularly hazardous, 96 percent of the workers were employed temporarily, with permanent employees making up the remainder. The nature of the job contract was heavily skewed in the other sections also: wet finishing work (84% and 16 percent respectively of temporary and permanent workers), dry finishing (89% and 11%), and miscellaneous work (94% and 6%).

Variables	Percentage (%)	Number (N)
Type of job within tannery occupation		
Beam house	8.4	24
Wet finishing	24.5	70
Dry finishing	50.4	142
Miscellaneous	16.7	48
Work experience in current tannery		
Up to 5 years	34.3	96
6 to 10 years	33.5	96
11 to 20 years	22.4	64
20+ years	9.8	28
Work experience in previous tannery		
Up to 5 years	43.4	43
6 to 10 years	38.4	38
11 to 20 years	13.1	13
20+ years	5.1	5
Type of job contract		
Temporary job (daily wages)	89.2	253
Permanent job	10.8	31
Working hours in day		
7 to 8 hours	47.2	134
9 to 10 hours	25.5	73
11 to 12 hours	27.3	77
Working days in a week		
Six days in a week	48.3	137
Seven days in a week	51.7	147
Total	**100.0**	**284**

Table 1.
Work related characteristics of tannery workers.

3.2 Awareness about the exposure of hazardous chemicals and work environment

Workers' awareness of hazards involve in tannery operation is presented in **Table 2**. About 79 percent of the workers in the age group of 16–24 years agreed with the statement that "tannery work is very hazardous in nature" found to be highest. Awareness of the above statement varies from 73 to 93 percent for the educational attainment, religion, caste, media exposure, and standard of living index among the tannery workers. It was found that tannery workers having a middle-school level of education were 3.01 times more likely to be aware of the hazards as compared to the illiterate or less educated ones. Those with a comparatively higher standard of living were 2.08 times more likely to agree that "tannery work is very hazardous in nature" than those having a lower standard of living. Agreement with the statement that "tannery workers work in the very hazardous work environment" ranges from 55 to 79 percent for the predictors such as age,

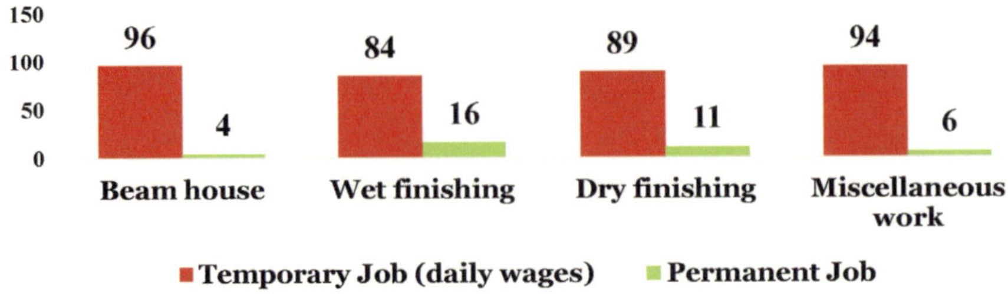

Figure 1.
Percent distribution of job contract by their type of work they usually do in tannery reported by tannery workers.

education, religion, caste, media exposure, and standard of living index. Tannery workers aged 36 and above were 0.34 times, and those who had a medium level of media exposure were 0.58 times less likely to aware of a hazardous work environment. We also examined the perceptions about exposure to hazardous chemicals in tanning processes. The awareness varied between 40 and 69 percent according to selected background variables. Odds ratio show that workers having a middle level of education were 0.43 times, and those with a medium level of media exposure are 0.54 times less likely to aware of the exposure of hazardous chemicals used in the tanning process. We also tried to understand the awareness of exposure to hazardous tissues involved in the tanning process. It was found that awareness ranged from 40 to 65 percent, depending on age, education, religion, caste, media exposure, and standard of living index. The odds ratio shows that tannery workers aged 36 years and above were 0.44 times less likely to aware of the hazardous tissues involved in the tanning process.

The awareness of potential health hazards involved in the tanning process by type of work is presented in **Table 3**. It is seen that 83 wet finishing and dry finishing (about 80%) workers were aware that the tannery work is hazardous. Similarly, 66 and 64 percent wet finishing and dry finishing workers engaged in tannery workers accepted that they worked in an unsafe work environment. Most of the workers (69%) in the wet finishing section reported that tannery workers were exposed to several hazardous chemicals during the tanning process, which was following by workers engaged in dry finishing (55%), Beam house work (50%), and workers engaged in miscellaneous work (49%). Around two-thirds of the workers involved in wet finishing were agreed that hazardous tissue engaged in the tanning process.

Awareness about the health hazard due to work in tannery occupation.

This research work examined awareness of health problems that may occur in tannery work. Various health issues like respiratory trouble, skin complaints, eye-related, and gastrointestinal issues were observed, which are presented in **Table 4**. Tannery workers who belong to the younger cohort (16–24 years) reported a higher awareness of respiratory problems (38%), skin complaints (59%), and gastrointestinal issues (21%) than those aged 36 years and above. There is an increasing awareness of educational attainment. Workers with high school education and more showed higher awareness of respiratory problems (52%), skin complaints (67%) in comparison to illiterate workers. Further, Hindu workers were more aware of respiratory problems (33%), skin complaints (55%), and gastrointestinal problems (16%) as compared to Muslim workers. Similarly, other caste group workers were also more aware of respiratory problems (29%), eye-related issues (46%), and the gastrointestinal problem (19%) compared to the schedule caste and other caste group workers.

Background Variables	Tannery work is very hazardous in nature		Tannery workers work in hazardous work environment		Tannery workers are exposed to many hazardous chemicals		Hazardous tissues involve in tanning process	
	Percent (%)	Odds CI	Percent (%)	Odds CI	Percent (%)	Odds CI	Percent (%)	Odds CI
Age in years								
16–24	79.3		79.3		68.9		65.5	
25–35	78.6	1.23 [0.42–3.65]	65.0	0.54 [0.20–1.49]	59.2	0.71 [0.28–1.78]	55.3	0.66 [0.27–1.62]
36+	74.3	0.89 [0.31–2.57]	55.2	0.34**[0.13–0.93]	52.6	0.55 [0.22–1.35]	46.0	0.44*[0.18–1.07]
Education								
Illiterate	73.8		59.3		57.7		50.8	
Up to primary	78.9	1.27 [0.52–3.12]	63.1	0.98 [0.46–2.10]	60.5	0.98 [0.46–2.09]	55.2	1.08 [0.51–2.28]
Middle school	88.0	3.01* [0.73–12.34]	60.0	0.94 [0.36–2.46]	40.0	0.43* [0.16–1.14]	40.0	0.66 [0.25–1.73]
High school & above	78.7	1.23 [0.40–3.79]	69.7	1.31 [0.49–3.49]	57.5	0.78 [0.30–2.00]	57.5	1.27 [0.50–3.23]
Religion								
Hindu	83.3		64.5		59.3		47.9	
Muslim	72.8	0.63 [0.31–1.26]	59.5	0.94 [0.53–1.66]	55.3	0.94 [0.53–1.66]	53.1	1.51 [0.86–2.66]
Caste								
Schedule caste	80.6		61.8		58.6		51.0	
Other backward class	65.3	0.41** [0.20–0.86]	59.6	0.80 [0.41–1.57]	63.4	1.14 [0.58–2.24]	61.5	1.31 [0.67–2.55]
Others	93.7	4.60 [0.56–37.80]	62.5	1.21[0.39–3.76]	50.0	0.84 [0.28–2.50]	50.0	0.92 [0.31–2.74]

Background Variables	Tannery work is very hazardous in nature		Tannery workers work in hazardous work environment		Tannery workers are exposed to many hazardous chemicals		Hazardous tissues involve in tanning process	
	Percent (%)	Odds CI	Percent (%)	Odds CI	Percent (%)	Odds CI	Percent (%)	Odds CI
Media exposure								
Low	76.9		64.6		61.5		53.8	
Medium	74.6	0.74 [0.35–1.59]	55.8	0.58* [0.30–1.11]	52.1	0.54* [0.28–1.03]	47.1	0.59 [0.31–1.12]
High	79.0	0.64 [0.22–1.77]	67.9	0.66 [0.28–1.57]	60.4	0.83 [0.35–1.97]	56.7	0.79 [0.34–1.85]
Standard of living index								
Low	73.8		56.0		52.3		46.7	
Medium	75.2	1.17 [0.58–2.39]	60.6	1.34 [0.73–2.49]	56.1	1.18 [0.64–2.18]	50.5	1.07 [0.58–1.98]
High	80.6	2.08* [0.92–4.72]	68.1	1.94* [0.98–3.81]	62.5	1.46 [0.75–2.83]	57.9	1.42 [0.74–2.75]
Total	**76.0**		**61.0**		**57.0**		**51.0**	

$^{*}p < 0.1$.
$^{**}p < 0.05$.

Table 2.
Awareness among the tannery workers about the involvement of hazards in tannery work by some selected background characteristics.

Statements	Beam house	Wet finishing	Dry finishing	Miscellaneous	Overall	(N)
Tannery work is very hazardous in nature						
Agree	62.5	82.9	80.4	61.7	51.4	217
Disagree	37.5	17.1	19.6	38.3	48.6	67
Tannery workers work in hazardous work environment						
Agree	58.3	65.7	63.6	48.9	56.7	174
Disagree	41.7	34.3	36.4	51.1	43.3	110
Tannery workers are exposed to many hazardous chemicals						
Agree	50.0	68.6	54.6	48.9	61.3	161
Disagree	50.0	31.4	45.5	51.1	38.7	123
Hazardous tissues involve in tanning process						
Agree	41.7	58.6	50.3	48.9	76.4	146
Disagree	58.3	41.4	49.7	51.1	23.6	138
Total	**100.0**	**100.0**	**100.0**	**100.0**	**100.0**	**284**

Table 3.
Awareness about the health hazard involved in tanning process by their type of work they usually do in tannery.

3.3. Qualitative measure of environmental exposure by type of work

The chemicals used in tanning processes are not consumed but discharged into the environment as effluents. Effluents contain organic matter, chromium, sulphides, and solid waste. Qualitative assessment of exposure at the workplace may be a useful tool for evaluating hazardous working conditions. **Table 5** presents qualitative measures of environmental exposure by different work categories. The results show that more than half (54%) of the workers engaged in beam housework followed by wet finishing (44%) and miscellaneous work (43%) had moderate to high exposure to chemicals. About one-third of Beamhouse workers (33%) and over a quarter (26%) of the wet finishing had moderate to high dermal contact with the chemicals. Further, 63 percent of the workers engaged in Beamhouse work, 51 percent doing miscellaneous work, 47 percent in wet finishing, and 36% in dry finishing reported exposure to dust. Furthermore, 50 percent of the beam house workers, 43 percent workers in wet finishing, 34 percent in miscellaneous work, and 30 percent in dry finishing had moderate to high exposure to ergonomic stressors.

3.4 Preventive measure and experiencing the different working condition

The preventive and safety measures appropriate for the work are presented in **Table 6**. The highest use of gloves and masks is seen in Beamhouse work (12 & 13% respectively), wet finishing (10 & 16%), miscellaneous (9 & 17%), and dry finishing (6.3 and 9%). Most tannery workers (69–92%), temporary as well as permanent, reported that they were involved in loading and unloading of raw hides manually in tannery premises. Only a small proportion (4.3–10%) used trolleys for loading and unloading. A substantial proportion of tannery workers had high exposure to humidity (69–88%), heat (69–84%), noise (78–87%). Additionally, most (51–63%) had become accustomed to the smell of hide. Most tannery workers also reported that exhaust fans (88–99%).

	Respiratory Problems		Skin Complaints		Eye related problems		Gastrointestinal problems	
Background Variables	**Percent (%)**	**Chi-square**	**Percent (%)**	**Chi-square**	**Percent (%)**	**Chi-square**	**Percent (%)**	**Chi-square**
Age in years								
16–24	37.9	$\chi 2 = 4.56$ $p < 0.335$	58.6	$\chi 2 = 1.76$ $p < 0.780$	24.1	$\chi 2 = 13.89$ $p < 0.008$	20.6	$\chi 2 = 2.19$ $p < 0.700$
25–35	25.2		53.4		34.9		13.5	
36+	23.6		53.9		38.1		12.5	
Education								
Illiterate	19.2	$\chi 2 = 19.48$ $p < 0.003$	54.5	$\chi 2 = 8.46$ $p < 0.206$	37.4	$\chi 2 = 4.47$ $p < 0.613$	11.7	$\chi 2 = 11.86$ $p < 0.065$
Up to primary	23.6		39.4		31.5		7.8	
Middle school	40.0		56.0		36.0		24.0	
High school & above	51.5		66.6		27.2		21.2	
Religion								
Hindu	33.3	$\chi 2 = 18.91$ $p < 0.000$	55.2	$\chi 2 = 1.14$ $p < 0.566$	22.9	$\chi 2 = 10.71$ $p < 0.005$	15.6	$\chi 2 = 1.11$ $p < 0.575$
Muslim	21.8		53.7		42.0		12.7	
Caste								
Schedule caste	22.5	$\chi 2 = 26.26$ $p < 0.000$	54.3	$\chi 2 = 7.65$ $p < 0.265$	34.4	$\chi 2 = 22.02$ $p < 0.001$	10.2	$\chi 2 = 24.80$ $p < 0.000$
Other backward class	28.8		57.6		46.1		19.2	
Others	12.5		62.5		6.25		0.0	
Media exposure								
Low	36.9	$\chi 2 = 23.45$ $p < 0.000$	61.5	$\chi 2 = 5.48$ $p < 0.241$	35.3	$\chi 2 = 6.67$ $p < 0.154$	21.5	$\chi 2 = 14.24$ $p < 0.007$
Medium	13.0		51.4		39.8		6.5	
High	38.2		53.0		28.4		19.7	

	Respiratory Problems		Skin Complaints		Eye related problems		Gastrointestinal problems	
Background Variables	**Percent (%)**	**Chi-square**	**Percent (%)**	**Chi-square**	**Percent (%)**	**Chi-square**	**Percent (%)**	**Chi-square**
Standard of living index								
Low	28.0	$\chi 2 = 5.47$	50.4	$\chi 2 = 3.47$	28.9	$\chi 2 = 5.16$	14.9	$\chi 2 = 9.34$
Medium	20.2	$p < 0.242$	53.9	$p < 0.483$	41.5	$p < 0.271$	11.2	$p < 0.053$
High	28.4		59.0		37.5		14.7	
Total	**25.7**		**54.2**		**35.5**		**13.7**	

Table 4.
Percent distribution of tannery workers who were aware about the health problems involve in tannery work.

	Beam house	Wet finishing	Dry finishing	Miscellaneous work	Chi-square	N
Chemicals in the Air[1]						
No exposure	25.0	24.3	30.1	17.0	$\chi2 = 8.09$ $p < 0.231$	74
Low exposure	20.8	31.4	37.1	40.4		99
Moderate/ High exposure	54.2	44.3	32.8	42.6		111
Dermal exposure to chemicals[2]						
No exposure	33.3	24.3	32.2	17.0	$\chi2 = 16.43$ $p < 0.012$	79
Low exposure	33.3	50.0	49.0	74.5		148
Moderate/ High exposure	33.4	25.7	18.8	8.5		57
Airborne dust[3]						
No exposure	25.0	21.4	34.3	17.0	$\chi2 = 12.28$ $p < 0.056$	78
Low exposure	12.5	31.4	29.3	31.9		82
Moderate/ High exposure	62.5	47.2	36.4	51.1		124
Ergonomic stressors[4]						
No exposure	20.8	18.6	37.1	19.2	$\chi2 = 14.15$ $p < 0.028$	80
Low exposure	29.2	38.6	32.8	46.8		103
Moderate/ High exposure	50.0	42.8	30.1	34.0		101
Total	**100.0**	**100.0**	**100.0**	**100.0**		**284**

[1]*Chemicals in the air (no exposure, low exposure, moderate exposure, high exposure, very high exposure) was based on qualitative rating of exposure assessment as [0] No exposure: no contact with agent, agent is used in workplace but is very unlikely to result in exposure to workers involved. [1] Low exposure: infrequent contact with agent at low concentrations, Agent is used in a closed/controlled system; there are no specific activities that enhance exposure; exposure takes place because of presence at the shop floor. [2] Moderate exposure: frequent contact with agent at low concentrations, Agent is used throughout the closed/controlled process and exposure mainly occurs by passive contact; infrequent contact is needed with the agent. [3] High exposure: Frequent contact with agent at high concentrations, Nature of the production process and associated manual activities makes regular contact necessary; agent causes exposure during manual activities and around particular sources such as presses, drums. [4] Very high exposure: Frequent contact with agent at very high concentrations, Agent is used in manual activities that introduce frequent peak exposures such as cleaning, opening a press, spraying paint.*

[2]*Dermal exposure to chemicals (no exposure, moderate exposure, high exposure) was based on qualitative rating of exposure assessment as [0] No skin contact: no contact with agent. [1] Moderate exposure: infrequent skin contact with agent contact occurs during specific activities that are not part of the daily work routine. [2] High exposure: frequent skin contact with agent regular contact is unavoidable due to particular activities in daily work practice.*

[3]*Another important variable airborne dust (no exposure, low exposure, moderate exposure, high exposure, very high exposure) was based on qualitative rating of exposure assessment as [0] No exposure: clear visibility. [1] Low exposure: visibility more than 10 m. [2] Moderate exposure: visibility between 5 to 10 m. [3] High exposure: visibility between 1 to 5 m. [4] Very high exposure: visibility less than 1 m.*

[4]*Ergonomic stressors (no exposure, low exposure, moderate exposure, high exposure, very high exposure) was based on qualitative rating of exposure assessment as [0] No exposure: does not occur (< 10% of work time). [1] Low exposure: less than 25% of daily work time. [2] Moderate exposure: 25–49% of daily work time. [3] High exposure: 50–74% of daily work time. [4] Very high exposure: 75% or more of daily work time. Exposure of waste water of chromium (no exposure, moderate exposure, high exposure) was based on qualitative rating of exposure assessment as [0] No exposure: no contact with chromium water. [1] Moderate exposure: infrequent contact with chromium water. [2] High exposure: frequent contact with chromium water.*

Table 5.
Qualitative measures of environmental exposure by their type of work among the tannery workers.

Variables	Beam house	Wet finishing	Dry finishing	Miscellaneous work	Overall	Number (N)
Use of glove						
Often	12.5	10.0	6.3	8.5	8.1	23
Sometimes	41.7	50.0	51.7	42.6	48.9	139
Never	45.8	40.0	42.0	48.9	43.0	122
Use of mask						
Often	12.5	15.7	9.0	17.0	12.3	35
Sometimes	29.2	48.6	49.0	42.6	46.1	131
Never	58.3	35.7	42.0	40.4	41.6	118
Involved in loading and unloading of raw hides manually						
Yes	91.7	90.0	69.2	87.2	79.2	225
No	8.3	10.0	30.8	12.8	20.8	59
Involved in loading and unloading of raw hides by trolley						
Yes	8.3	8.6	9.8	4.3	8.5	24
No	91.7	91.4	90.2	95.7	91.5	260
Feeling humidity in tannery premises						
Yes	87.5	84.3	68.5	72.3	74.7	212
No	12.5	15.7	31.5	27.7	25.3	72
Feeling heat in tannery premises						
Yes	79.2	84.3	69.2	80.8	75.7	215
No	20.8	15.7	30.8	19.2	24.3	69
Feeling extreme noise in tannery premises						
Yes	83.3	87.1	78.3	85.1	82.0	233
No	16.7	12.9	21.7	14.9	18.0	51
Comfortable with smell of hides						
Yes	62.5	51.4	54.6	53.2	54.2	154
No	37.5	48.6	45.5	46.8	45.8	130
Exhaustive fan						
Yes	87.5	98.6	96.5	95.7	96.3	273
No	12.5	1.4	3.5	4.3	3.7	11
Total	**100.0**	**100.0**	**100.0**	**100.0**	**100.0**	**284**

Table 6.
Percentage of tannery workers who use preventive measures and experienced different environmental conditions in tannery premises by their type of work.

4. Discussion

The results from this study of male tannery workers revealed that the workers were exposed to chemicals, leather dust, which contains chromium, and physical hazards. A substantial proportion of the tannery workers reported awareness of the health risks of the various tanning processes. The physical and cognitive difficulty levels of the job in tanneries were like previous studies [8–10]. It is essential to mention here that there are very few studies conducted on tannery workers in the Indian context.

The results of our study validate the need for further efforts to minimize hazardous occupational health risks among tannery workers. However, findings depict tannery workers aged 36 years & above are less likely to be aware of the hazardous work environment, and malignant tissues involved in the tanning process, lack of protective equipment and safety devices showed a significant double risk for occupational health and injuries [11–14]. **Previous findings** agree with a study on salt workers found that there is a considerable gap between their knowledge and practices, along with protective measures [15]. Furthermore, a study conducted on chronic conditions, workplace safety, and job demands in Colorado revealed that non-provision of workplace safety led to employees' chronic health conditions and contributed to absenteeism and poor job performance. It also influences the physical and cognitive difficulties of the workers associated with the work [16]. Other factors also significantly affect the perceptions of health risks: age, education, religion, caste, media exposure, and standard of living index. Workers reported that they are aware that they have the chance of getting respiratory problems, skin complaints, eye-related, and gastrointestinal problems from the tannery. A substantial proportion of workers experienced severe conditions, such as humidity (69–88% of those surveyed), heat (69–84%), noise (78–87%); they had also got used to the smell of hides (51–63%). Comparable outcomes found by a study led in some developing countries concentrating on the upshot of work-related acquaintance to noise and heat on the health of the workers. Results portray that those who worked in the foundry had high thermal stress, high noise levels, high visual defects, high muscle cramps problem, high visual disability and describe non-use of protective equipment and poor occupational hygiene and safety measures were also affected the health problem among workers [17–20]. Our study recommended that leather dust exposure be reduced by providing gloves and masks and by installing a hood duct to provide better ventilation and removal of leather dust from the work area as also recommended by previous researches [21].

This research also suggested risks should be assessed for their potential consequences on health. Liquid effluents contain organic matter, chromium, sulfides, and solid wastes. A qualitative assessment of exposure showed that moderate to high exposure to chemicals and also contacted them. It has been reported from the literature that the workers on exposure to leather dust, which contains chromium in the protein-bound form, exhibited a higher mean concentration of urinary and blood chromium [8]. The workers engaged in beam housework, miscellaneous work, wet finishing, and dry finishing also reported moderate to high exposure to dust and ergonomic stressors. The use of safety gear was the highest in beam housework, followed by wet finishing, miscellaneous work, and dry finishing. This study also recognized a lack of awareness of the health risks in tannery operations and shortcomings in the use of preventive measures. Employers must raise awareness of health risks and ensure compliance with safety measures. But at the same time, qualitative results of focused group discussion with workers from small scale industries in Tanzania show high levels (>90%) of self-reported exposure to health problems, and low use of protective measures [22]. In continuation of the previous findings, a case study of electroplating sector workers in the United Kingdom showed that the employees had sound knowledge of the hazardous nature of chemicals used at the workplace [23].

An intervention study focused on prevention of work-related skin problems assessed the occupational health and safety among wet workers. The study found significant behavior change and fewer skin problems among workers in the intervention group as compared to the control group. The intervention was successful in enhancing knowledge and changing behavior [24]. Literature suggests most workers had an essential awareness of the existence of occupational health and safety legislation, but they were unaware of their legal responsibilities. They were found to have minimal occupational and safety training [25–29].

5. Conclusion

The findings of this study reveal that the tannery workers work in a very hazardous work environment and susceptible to health risks. Although, tannery workers are less aware of the health hazard involved in the tanning process and even not aware of the exposure to hazardous chemicals at the work place. Evidence from the qualitative measures of environmental exposure pointed out that they work in different activities at the tannery and having different exposures. Further, the study findings reveal that tannery workers are not utilizing the appropriate preventive measures as per the protocol. The outcomes of the study give a clear indication of the effect of the workstation environment on the health status of workers and require the use of adequate measures to improve the facilities and thereby the health status of tannery workers.

Declarations

Ethics approval and consent to participate

We have received ethical approval from the board. The Student Research Ethics Committee approved the study of the International Institute for Population Sciences Mumbai, India. We have also obtained consent to participate from each of the respondents before starting the interview. The confidentiality of information has been maintained.

Consent for publication

Not applicable.

Availability of supporting data

This research is based on primary data.

Funding

Not received any funding.

Authors' contributions

GCK developed the questionnaire, collected the data, contributed in acquisition of data. SKS PC conceived and designed the experiments. GCK PC analyzed the data. GCK PC wrote the manuscript. SKS critically revised the draft.

Abbreviations

ILO	International Labour Organization
WHO	World Health Organizations
DALY	disability adjusted life years
PPS	probability proportional to size
OR	odds ratio
CI	confidence interval

Author details

Gyan Chandra Kashyap[1*], Praveen Chokhandre[2] and Shri Kant Singh[3]

1 Institute of Health Management Research, Bangalore, India

2 GEH, International Institute for Population Sciences, Deonar, Mumbai, India

3 Department of Mathematical Demography and Statistics, International Institute for Population Sciences, Deonar, Mumbai, India

*Address all correspondence to: gyan.ck@iihmrbangalore.edu.in

References

[1] International Labour Organization (ILO). Occupational safety and health (OSH). 2019. https://www.ilo.org/moscow/areas-of-work/occupational-safety-and- ealth/WCMS_249278/lang--en/index.htm.

[2] World Health Organization. Occupation Health. 2019.https://www.who.int/topics/occupational_health/en/

[3] Neira, M. Towards a healthier future of work (WHO). 2019. https://www.ilo.org/safework/events/safeday/33thinkpieces/WCMS681618/lang--en/index.htm

[4] Neira M, Pfeiffer M, Campbell-Lendrum D, Prüss-Ustün A. Towards a healthier and safer environment. The Lancet. 2018 Feb 3;391(10119):408-10.

[5] Prüss-Ustün A, van Deventer E, Mudu P, Campbell-Lendrum D, Vickers C, Ivanov I, Forastiere F, Gumy S, Dora C, Adair-Rohani H, Neira M. Environmental risks and non-communicable diseases. Bmj. 2019 Jan 28;364.

[6] World Health Organization. Healthy environments: why do the matter and what can we do?. World Health Organization. 2019.

[7] World Health Organization (WHO). The world health report 2002: reducing risks, promoting healthy life. 2002

[8] Rastogi SK, Pandey A, Tripathi S. Occupational health risks among the workers employed in leather tanneries at Kanpur. Indian journal of occupational and environmental medicine. 2008 Dec;12(3):132.

[9] Arunkumar Yogaraj G, Ravi R. Impact of workplace environment on health of leather factory workers. International Journal of Community Medicine and Public Health. 2017 Aug;4(8):2674.

[10] Islam R, Hossain MS, Siddique MA. Occupational health hazards and safety practices among the workers of tannery industry in Bangladesh. Jahangirnagar University Journal of Biological Sciences. 2017 Aug 27;6(1):13-22.

[11] Bull N, Riise T, Moen BE. Work-related injuries and occupational health and safety factors in smaller enterprises—a prospective study. Occupational Medicine. 2002 Mar 1;52(2):70-4.

[12] Hämäläinen P, Saarela KL, Takala J. Global trend according to estimated number of occupational accidents and fatal work-related diseases at region and country level. Journal of safety research. 2009 Jan 1;40(2):125-39.

[13] Takala J, Hämäläinen P, Saarela KL, Yun LY, Manickam K, Jin TW, Heng P, Tjong C, Kheng LG, Lim S, Lin GS. Global estimates of the burden of injury and illness at work in 2012. Journal of occupational and environmental hygiene. 2014 May 4;11(5):326-37.

[14] Turkkan A, Pala K. Trends in occupational injuries and fatality in Turkey. International journal of occupational safety and ergonomics. 2016 Oct 1;22(4):457-62.

[15] Haldiya KR, Sachdev R, Mathur ML, Saiyed HN. Knowledge, attitude and practices related to occupational health problems among salt workers working in the desert of Rajasthan, India. Journal of occupational health. 2005;47(1):85-8.

[16] Jinnett K, Schwatka N, Tenney L, Brockbank CV, Newman LS. Chronic conditions, workplace safety, and job demands contribute to absenteeism and job performance. Health Affairs. 2017 Feb 1;36(2):237-44.

[17] Gomes J, Lloyd OL, Revitt DM. The influence of personal protection, environmental hygiene and exposure to pesticides on the health of immigrant farm workers in a desert country. International archives of occupational and environmental health. 1999 Jan 1;72(1):40-5.

[18] Gomes J, Lloyd O, Norman N. The health of the workers in a rapidly developing country: effects of occupational exposure to noise and heat. Occupational medicine. 2002 May 1;52(3):121-8.

[19] Hubbard R. Occupational dust exposure and the aetiology of cryptogenic fibrosing alveolitis. European Respiratory Journal. 2001 Jul 1;18(32 suppl):119s–21s.

[20] Chandrasekaran V, Dilara K, Padmavathi R. Pulmonary functions in tannery workers--a cross sectional study. Indian journal of physiology and pharmacology. 2014 Jul 1;58(3):206-10.

[21] Thepaksorn P, Thongjerm S, Incharoen S, Siriwong W, Harada K, Koizumi A. Job safety analysis and hazard identification for work accident prevention in para rubber wood sawmills in southern Thailand. Journal of occupational health. 2017:16-0204.

[22] Rongo LM, Barten FJ, Msamanga GI, Heederik D, Dolmans WM. Occupational exposure and health problems in small-scale industry workers in Dar es Salaam, Tanzania: a situation analysis. Occupational Medicine. 2004 Jan 1;54(1):42-6.

[23] Sadhra S, Petts J, McAlpine S, Pattison H, MacRae S. Workers' understanding of chemical risks: electroplating case study. Occupational and environmental medicine. 2002 Oct 1;59(10):689-95.

[24] Held E, Mygind K, Wolff C, Gyntelberg F, Agner T. Prevention of work related skin problems: an intervention study in wet work employees. Occupational and Environmental Medicine. 2002 Aug 1;59(8):556-61.

[25] Fonteyn PN, Olsberg D, Cross JA. Small business owners' knowledge of their occupational health and safety (OHS) legislative responsibilities. International Journal of Occupational Safety and Ergonomics. 1997 Jan 1;3(1-2):41-57.

[26] Salvador LR, Van Thinh D. Occupational Safety and Health: An overview. In2016 IEEE 11th International Symposium on Applied Computational Intelligence and Informatics (SACI) 2016 May 12 (pp. 355-360). IEEE.

[27] Walters DR. Preventive Services in Occupational Health and Safety in Europe: Developments and trends in the 1990s. International journal of health services. 1997 Apr;27(2):247-71.

[28] Collinson DL. Surviving the rigs': safety and surveillance on North Sea oil installations. Organization studies. 1999 Jul;20(4):579-600.

[29] Isaksson K, Hellgren J, Pettersson P. Repeated downsizing: Attitudes and well-being for surviving personnel in a Swedish retail company. InHealth effects of the new labour market 2002 (pp. 85-101). Springer, Boston, MA.

Section 2

Physiological and Psychosocial Wellbeing

Chapter 7

Muscle Health: The Gateway to Population Health Management

Thomas Gilliam and Paul Terpeluk

Abstract

The muscle on your frame is a prime indicator of health and longevity. Dr. Paul Terpeluk with the Cleveland Clinic has stated that muscular strength is the new vital sign of workplace health and safety. Research studies focusing on Type II diabetes, cardiovascular disease, musculo-skeletal injuries, certain cancers and the delay of dementia have shown a strong correlation between disease prevention and muscular strength. IPCS' database of over 500,000 strength tests have shown a workers' absolute strength today is at least 14% weaker than the worker 15 years ago and weighs about 8 pounds more. Over the last 10 years, there has been a significant shift by 52% with an increase in the number of workers with a BMI of 35 or greater. The Cleveland Clinic implemented a new hire muscular strength assessment to place new hire applicants into jobs that match their physical capability in 2011. The outcomes show a statistically significant reduction in number of employee health, pharmacy and workers' compensation claims and costs with overall savings near $25 million. Musculo-skeletal health of the worker can be improved. When a worker maintains good muscular strength, the worker is more productive, has fewer medical claims and workers' compensation claims.

Keywords: muscle health, muscle strength, musculo-skeletal, disease prevention, cost savings

1. Introduction

Population Health continues to expand especially as new research demonstrates ways to better manage a person's health. One area of interest is the impact muscle has on enhancing health and disease prevention [1–12]. A healthy and strong muscle mass increases the chance of better managing and preventing certain diseases such as Type II diabetes, cardiovascular disease, certain cancers, dementia and hypertension to name a few [3–5]. A healthy muscle mass also helps in maintaining a healthier body weight, the ability to sustain an adequate overall body metabolism with age and an enhanced immune system to help fight off various viruses and disease [6, 8, 9]. Muscular strength with aging puts individuals at greater risk for sarcopenia (loss of muscle) not only for the diseases already mentioned by also for slips, falls, functionality and frailty [4, 11–12].

2. Research general

In 2006, Wolfe discussed the underappreciated role of muscle in health and disease [1]. He discussed the importance of future research to include factors related to muscle mass, strength and metabolic syndrome. Wolfe focused on the importance of muscle protein and the pool of amino acids in maintaining a relatively constant plasma glucose concentration. He also discussed the role muscle plays in obesity and Type II diabetes. Argiles and associates in 2016 supports Wolfe's research on the importance of muscle regulating protein metabolism throughout the body [4]. Both of these studies strongly support maintaining a healthy and strong muscle mass throughout one's lifespan especially to prevent sarcopenia and certain diseases. This was further emphasized by Mrowka and Westphal in their article on "skeletal muscle in the fight against chronic disease" published in 2018 [5]. DeCarvalho and associates showed an inverse relationship between skeletal muscle mass adjusted for weight and BMI with metabolic syndrome in both males and females [2]. Their study researched 689 adults between the ages of 20–59. Mesinovic and associates discussed the connection between sarcopenia and Type II diabetes [10]. The loss of muscle alters glucose uptake in the muscle leading to more glucose in the blood which increases the risk of Type II diabetes.

2.1 Research sarcopenia

Sarcopenia is a critical concern not just because of the loss of muscle and its ability to fight disease and infection, but because the individual is at greater risk for slips, falls and injury [4, 11–16]. If not remedied, the loss of muscle can lead to a frail state which can be fatal [4]. Every day functionality and daily activities become more difficult to perform with the loss of muscle. Muscle protein breaks down and rebuilds daily. Sarcopenia can start as early age of 25 and accelerates after age 60 years and sometimes sooner. The inability to rebuild muscle protein as the body ages contributes to sarcopenia. It should be noted that as the body loses muscle, the loss of muscle strength (dynapenia) occurs more rapidly. It also should be noted that obese individuals are at greater risk for sarcopenia.

2.2 Research inflammation

Inflammation is associated with most chronic diseases [8, 9, 17]. There is compelling evidence that shows physical activity to include strength training offers a defense to chronic diseases. David Nieman discussed the link between physical activity and the body's immune system [9]. While there is compelling evidence to suggest that physical exercise will enhance the body's immune system, there is also evidence that suggests lengthy, intense workout sessions might be harmful to the body's immune system. Nieman suggests physical activity workouts should be no more than 60-minutes at a moderate-vigorous intensity to safely enhance the immune system [9].

2.3 Research cancer

One area of research that has increased dramatically focuses on muscle mass and strength related to cancer treatment and prevention [18–28]. Caan and associates in 2018 showed that women with non-metastatic breast cancer had 41% better chance of surviving with a healthier muscle mass compared to sarcopenic non-metastatic breast cancer patients [18]. The American College of Sports Medicine (ACSM) has published research showing the impact physical activity has in lowering the risk of at least 7 different cancers and increasing survivability [22–24, 26, 27]. ACSM recommends a variety of physical activities to include resistance training (strength), aerobic and balance with options for light, moderate or vigorous intensity. The

ACSM and the National Academy of Sports Medicine certify health and exercise professionals to work directly with cancer patients to improve their strength and muscle mass.

2.4 Research mortality

There is evidence demonstrating muscular strength as a predictor of mortality in a healthy population [29–34]. A meta-analysis by Garcia-Hermosa and colleagues show that individuals with good upper body and lower body strength have lower risk of mortality regardless of age [29]. ACSM has published numerous research studies demonstrating the effectiveness of resistance training on health for individuals from 15 to 90 plus years old [22–24, 26, 27]. Moberg recently published data about the significance of a "muscle memory" found in each myonucleous [30]. This study focused on how much impact does resistance training when done earlier in life has on muscle later in life. It appears that if resistance training was done earlier in life that your muscle will *retrain faster* in terms of regaining strength compared to if you are just beginning. The research is new and so there are many unanswered questions such as how much faster will strength return, will it return to previous strength levels and how long does the "muscle memory" retain previous strength levels? But the research also shows that it is never too late in life to reap the benefits of resistance training. Research shows the human body is able increase strength levels at any age – even those individuals in their 80's and 90's [22–24, 26, 27]. This is extremely important in preventing sarcopenia which can lead to frailty as well as cachexia which occurs with some diseases such as cancer [4, 28].

2.5 Research industrial worker

Despite the incredible abundance of research showing how a healthy muscle mass leads to a healthier lifestyle, the worker today in general is weaker and heavier than the worker 25 years ago. One reason for this is that physical demands of many jobs have been decreased due to robots and other ergonomic assists [35, 36]. Automation is good, especially in industry. It contributes to a safer workplace. But automation greatly diminishes the physical demands of the job which has impacted the overall health of the industrial worker.

Since 1960, the percentage of moderate intensity physically demanding jobs in the United States has decreased from about 50% to 20% in 2010, but the light intensity jobs have increased from 38% to about 55% [35]. Sedentary jobs increased as well from 15–22%. Most of these changes took place because of automation. This means the amount of physical work done by today's worker has greatly diminished.

Unfortunately, the less physically active the worker becomes, the greater the risk for injury and certain diseases. Some of this increased risk occurs because of an increase in body weight (fat weight) tied to the loss of muscle mass and strength.

3. IPCS

Industrial Physical Capability Services, Inc. (dba IPCS) performs muscular strength assessments for industry in the United States using isokinetic equipment for shoulder and knee flexion and extension at 60 degrees per second [37, 38]. Between 2005 and 2019, 406,731 strength tests were completed (327,913 males and 78,818 females). To compare changes in muscular strength, an analysis was made comparing the year 2005 to 2019 (a 15-year span).

Descriptive data for males and females (Means ± SD)						
	Female			Male		
	2005	2019	Kolmogorov–Smirnov Test	2005	2019	Kolmogorov–Smirnov Test
Age (yrs)	34.1 ± 10.34	33.8 ± 11.72	>.001	34.0 ± 10.34	34.1 ± 11.63	>.001
Height (in)	64.8 ± 2.94	64.3 ± 64.34	<.001	70.3 ± 2.99	71.0 ± 3.03	<.001
Weight (lbs)	167.8 ± 41.48	177.3 ± 47.92	<.001	205 ± 44.01	207.6 ± 49.50	<.001
BMI	28.1 ± 6.65	30.1 ± 7.59	<.001	29.1 ± 5.66	29.8 ± 6.57	<.001
Sample Size	2637	6701		23,274	13,219	

Table 1.
Physical characteristics and sample size (mean ± SD).

Knee and shoulder strength measures for males and females (Means ± SD)						
	Female			Male		
Absolute Strength	**2005**	**2019**	**Kolmogorov–Smirnov Test**	**2005**	**2019**	**Kolmogorov–Smirnov Test**
Shoulder (ft. pds)	102 ± 26.32	90 ± 25.74	<.001	189 ± 43.26	170 ± 43.27	<.001
Knee (ft. pds)	246 ± 81.76	235 ± 76.50	<.001	388 ± 89.23	347 ± 91.69	<.001

Table 2.
Absolute strength measures for the knee and shoulders (means ± SD).

Table 1 shows the physical characteristics of those new hire industrial applicants tested in 2005 compared to 2019 based on gender. Due to unequal sample sizes and unequal variances, the Kolmogorov–Smirnov Test was used to test for significance within gender between 2005 and 2019. There was no significant difference for age (>.001) within gender between 2005 and 2019. Height, weight and BMI was significantly different within gender between the two time periods. The female body weight increased most between 2005 and 2019 (+9.5 pounds). The BMI increased for both genders.

Changes in the absolute strength of the shoulder and knee flexors and extensors of the worker by age group between 2005 and 2019 is shown in **Table 2**. The absolute shoulder strength and knee strength decreased significantly (<.001) between 2005 and 2019 for males and females.

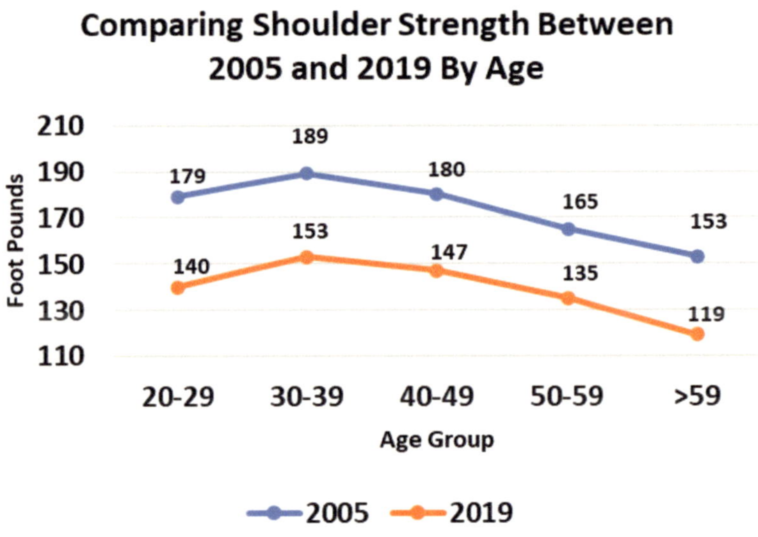

Figure 1.
Changes in absolute shoulder strength (ft. pds.) of the worker by age group.

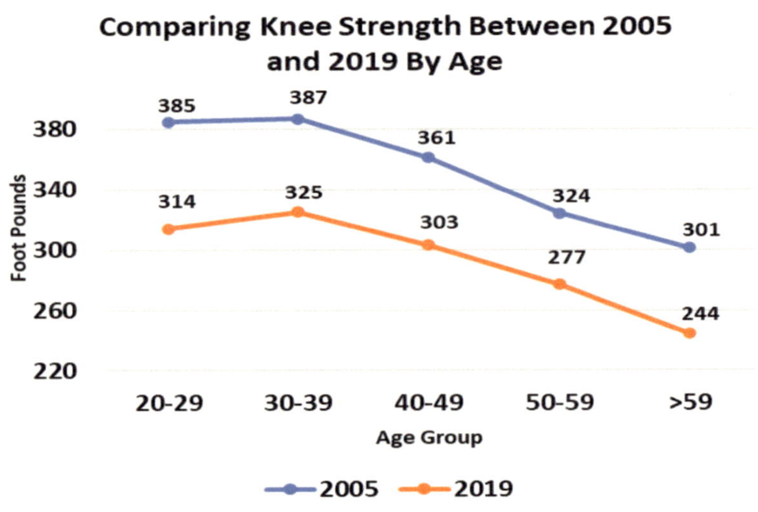

Figure 2.
Changes in absolute knee strength (ft. pds.) of the worker by age group.

Changes in the absolute strength of the shoulder and knee flexors and extensors of the worker by age group between 2005 and 2019 are shown in **Figures 1** and **2**, respectively.

Figure 1 shows for each age group that the shoulder strength is anywhere from 14.5% to 18.9% weaker in 2019 compared to 2005.

Figure 2 shows for each age group the absolute knee strength is anywhere from 18.2% to 22.2% weaker in 2019 compared to 2005. Both **Figures 1** and **2** show substantial difference in the strength of the worker between 2005 and 2019. **Figure 3** shows the differences between years by age groups as a percent change.

The first three figures show the absolute shoulder and knee strength has decreased on average by 18% across all age groups between 2005 and 2019. The figures also show after the 40–49 age group there is a rapid decrease in absolute

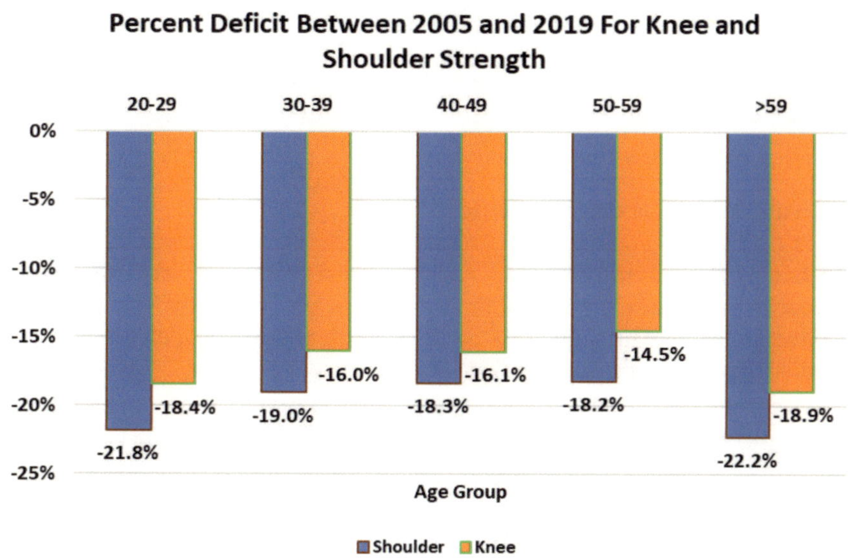

Figure 3.
Percent deficit in shoulder and knee strength between 2005 and 2019.

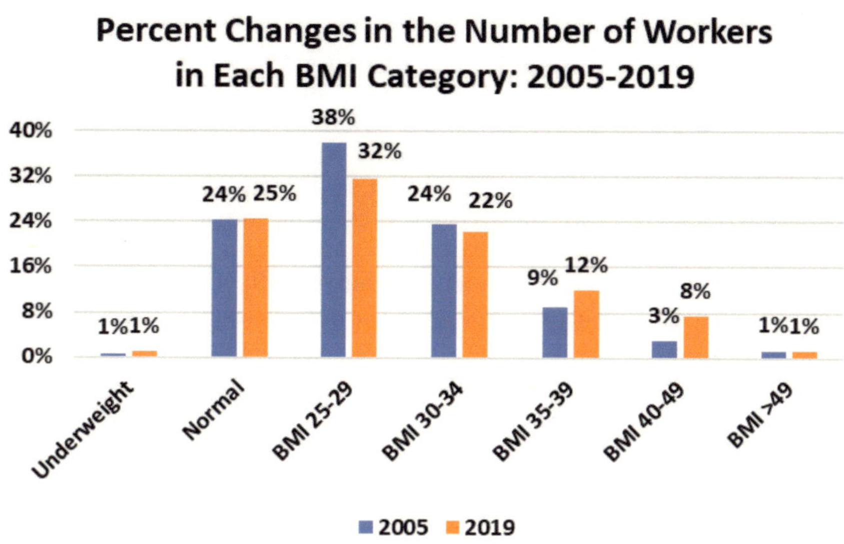

Figure 4.
Percent changes in number of Workers for each BMI category.

strength which supports the concept of loss of muscle mass and strength with aging along with an increase in sedentary lifestyles. Interestingly, the youngest age group (20–29) had the greatest deficit for the shoulder and knee strength when compared to the three age groups between 30 and 59. This is a reflection on the sedentary lifestyles found in children and youth which then carries over into industry.

During the IPCS testing process, height (in) and weight (pds) are measured. For research purposes IPCS calculates Body Mass Index (BMI) to monitor trends in obesity within the workplace. **Figure 4** compares the changes in the percent number of workers in each BMI category from 2005 to 2019. IPCS looks at changes in BMI for the category 50 or more or extreme morbid obesity. When comparing 2005 to 2019, the overweight category (BMI 25–30) decreased from 38–32% whereas the BMI categories equal to severe obesity (BMI 35 or more) and greater increased from 13.6% to 20.7% which represents a 52.2% increase. It is these higher BMI categories associated with an increase in certain diseases such as Type II diabetes, hypertension and cardiovascular disease. Further, work by Ostebye in 2007 has shown that those workers with a BMI of 35 or more have 2 times the number of soft tissue injuries, 7 times the workers' compensation costs and 13 times more lost work days [39].

4. Research study Cleveland clinic

IPCS has been involved providing a comprehensive strength screening evaluation for the new hires for the Cleveland Clinic since January 2011 [40]. This has resulted in the collection of new hire data related to strength and medical claims which have been studied from 2011 through 2017.

4.1 Research study design

This quasi-experimental, non-randomized study was conducted at Cleveland Clinic in northeast Ohio. It was designed to assess the impact of a strength screening assessment for nurses used at the time of hire, and compare the difference in health plan costs to newly employed nurses who did not receive the strength screening. Participants were identified from the applicant pool as part of the new hire process from January 2008 through December 2017. Applicants were either registered nurses, licensed vocational nurses, licensed practical nurses, or patient care nursing assistants applying for a nursing position in any unit of the hospital. The interviewing process for potential candidates consisted of an online application, followed by a phone interview and then an in-person interview if warranted. Nurses that passed these initial requirements for selection were then scheduled for a physical exam and a drug screen. A strength assessment screening was added to the existing hiring protocol as the last segment of the interview process for nurses hired from January 2011 through December 2017.

Nurses hired in January 2008 through December 2010, prior to the strength assessment screening implementation, served as a Historical Comparison Group. There were no significant environmental or business practice changes observed during this time period from January 2008 through December 2017, and health plan coverage did not change across the two time frames. The only difference in the selection process in 2011–2017 compared to 2008–2010 was the addition of the physical capability evaluation (PCE™). The project was overseen by hospital administrators, and conducted based on quality improvement protocols. Given that this was a retrospective analysis of a hiring practice policy, and not a formal research study, Institutional Review Board approval or research consent was not required.

The strength screening was conducted through an objective physical capability evaluation (PCE™). The PCE is designed to measure the applicant's isokinetic force generating capability (strength) of muscle groups based on the outcomes of a defensible job task analysis (JTA) [37]. The JTA was conducted according to guidelines of the Americans with Disabilities Act of 1990 (ADA) to determine the skills necessary to safely and effectively perform the essential functions associated with the nursing duties (e.g., lifting, carrying, bending, stooping, climbing, etc.). These validation studies were used to identify appropriate cut-off scores using the U.S. Department of Labor strength definitions for medium, heavy and very heavy job tasks [41]. It was determined that the "target score" for the nursing job category would be set at the medium strength level. The results of the JTA indicated that movement patterns of the major muscle groups involved with shoulder flexion and extension and knee flexion and extension were critical to safely performing the essential functions of the nursing jobs.

The PCE testing was conducted in the Occupational Medicine department, in a controlled environment using isokinetic equipment and a standardized testing process (tested at 60 degrees per second, two sets of five repetitions flexion and extension for knees and shoulders) administered by trained professionals [38]. To improve reliability of the measure, health system physical therapists and athletic instructors were trained and observed for proper technique administering the PCE, verifying that they completed the evaluation correctly. PCE results were collected at the time of conducting the assessment, and submitted to a centralized database for data interpretation. These objective evaluations were then interpreted by IPCS (a third party company). The interpretation included isokinetic measurements through:

1. a force curve analysis in which the applicant's force curves generated were compared to an unmatched normative force curve derived from nearly 500,000 normative curves in the existing database;

2. a body muscle symmetry analysis which involved comparing the applicant's right and left shoulder and knee scores, agonist to antagonist muscle groups and upper and lower body scores to a normative database consisting of more than 500,000 normative symmetry scores;

3. assessing the applicant's strength to body weight ratio score.

The screening took approximately 30 minutes to complete per applicant.

PCE data were analyzed based on proprietary algorithms, and scores were electronically returned to Human Resources through summary reports [37]. An applicant was recommended for hire if the PCE strength screening score was equal to or greater than the "target score".

4.2 Research study data sources and analysis

Medical claims cost data for the first 12-months of employment were obtained for each annual cohort from the employer-sponsored health plan. The analyses include data for all newly hired nurses that have 12-months of continuous enrollment in the employer-sponsored health plan after their hire date.

Total annual and per employee per month (PEPM) paid medical costs were calculated for nurses hired in each of the three years prior to initiation of the PCE (2008–2010), as well as for nurses hired after the PCE program was initiated (2011–2017).

4.3 Research study results

Of the 16,113 nurses who were included in this study, 85% were females and 15% were males. There were no refusals to take the physical capability screening.

Table 3 shows the number of eligible nurses hired in each group. There were 2481 eligible nurses hired in 2008–2010 in the Historical Comparison Group, and 13,632 eligible nurses in the PCE Group. The total member months for the Historical Comparison Group was 15,788 months, and for the PCE™ Group the total was 34,102 as shown in **Table 3**.

Figure 5 shows what percent of the new hires had medical claims for each group. The Historical group had significantly higher percentage of claims for those hired (57.4%) compared to those hired in the PCE group (28.4%).

As shown in **Table 4**, the difference for Average Medical Paid and the PEPM between the Historical Comparison Group and the PCE™ Group is $882 and $77.07, respectively. Due to unequal sample sizes and unequal variances, the Kolmogorov–Smirnov Test was used to test for significance between the Historical Comparison Group and the PCE Group.

The costs to implement the PCE™ program for 2011–2017 were $1,192,672. To calculate the savings for medical claim costs, the average claim cost for Historical group was multiplied by the number of new hires for the PCE group (13,632) times the percentage of new hire applicants that had a claim for the Historical group (57.4%) which is $22,519,682 (**Table 5**). The actual medical claim cost for the PCE group was $7,722,524. The combination of a smaller percentage of claims for the PCE group along with the lower average medical claim cost resulted in $14,797,158

	Historical group	PCE group
Number Hired	2481	13,632
Number Medical Claims	1425	3869
Number Member Months	15,788	34,102

Table 3.
The number of new hires, medical claims and member months for each group.

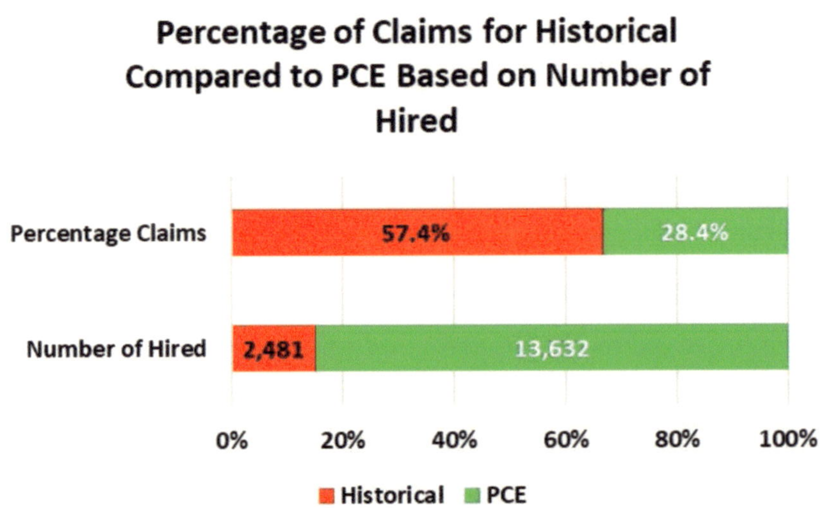

Figure 5.
Percentage of claims for each group based on number of new hires.

	Average Medical Claim Cost Mean ± SD	Per Empl Per Month Mean ± SD	Kolmogorov–Smirnov Test
Historical Group	$2878 ± 6930.73	$239.80 ± 577.49	<.001
PCE Group	$1996 ± 4836.42	$165.73 ± 399.53	<.001

Table 4.
Comparing average medical claim and PEPM costs between historical and PCE groups (means ± SD).

	Total Medical Costs
No PCE	$22,519,682
W/PCE	$7,722,524
Savings	$14,797,158

Table 5.
Total savings resulting from the PCE program.

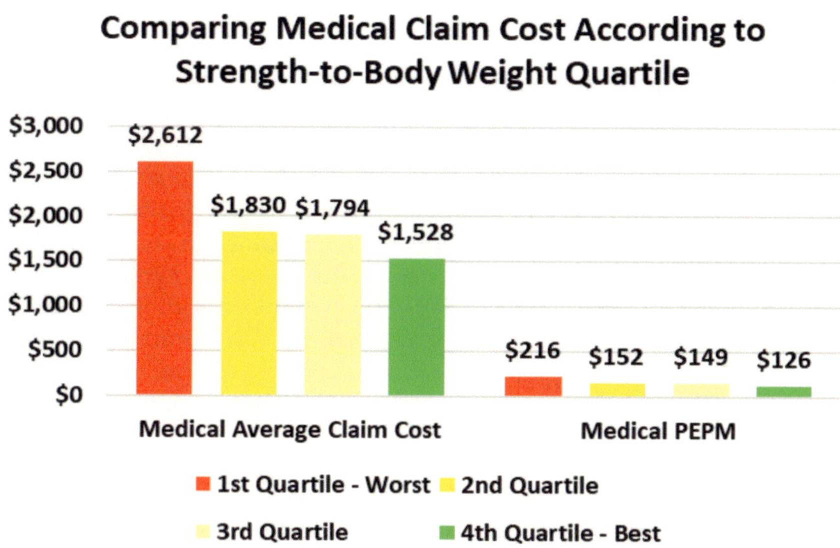

Figure 6.
Comparing medical claim costs for nurses based on quartile measures.

in savings between 2011 and 2017 (**Table 5**). The return on investment for the program was $12.41.

The combination of increased fat weight and loss of muscular strength results in a substantial decrease in the worker's strength to body weight ratio (SBW). (A worker's strength should be proportionate to his/her body weight.) It is clear that workers with a healthy strength to body weight ratio perform better, are safer and have fewer employee health claim costs. An analysis of the Cleveland Clinic SBW data shows that those nurses with the lower SBW scores (1st Quartile) medical costs were about 42% more compared to those nurses with a higher SBW score (4th Quartile) as shown in **Figure 6**. A non-parametric test computed the statistical differences between the four quartiles. A Kolmogorov–Smirnov Test was used to test for significance between the first and fourth quartile which was significant at the .001 level (**Figure 6**).

Those individuals in the lower quartile have either weak absolute strength and/or excess body weight compared to those who are in the upper quartile who have good absolute strength and a health body weight. The SBW is a good measure and predictor of health and injury risk. The SBW also shows the importance of maintain a healthy muscle mass and healthy body weight throughout life.

4.4 Research study conclusions

The Cleveland Clinic study shows that it is possible to design a defensible strength test to be used in the selection process for physically demanding nursing jobs. This study shows the importance of physical strength specifically in the nursing profession. When a nurse's physical capability is correctly matched to the physical demands of the job, a nurse can better meet the essential functions of the job and better serve patients. Also, the analysis of this study shows it is possible to hire through a work justified strength screening program a healthier worker who will have lower paid average medical and per employee per month costs in the first year of benefit eligibility. The results of this study support the premise that strength is a new vital sign of workplace health.

5. Conclusions

As automation continues to improve in the workplace and with fewer physically demanding jobs, the industrial worker will need to rely on means other than work to maintain a healthy and strong muscle mass. Without a resistance training intervention, the worker will continue to become weaker and heavier putting the worker at greater risk for injury and disease. This will lead to greater costs and absenteeism. How much of a responsibility will the employer have in providing such intervention programs remains to be seen. The intervention could be in short durations (10 minutes) several times a day at the workplace or providing some incentive to reimburse memberships at fitness centers. This is nothing new and it has not been very successful in the past. But making muscle health tied into a health/benefit deductible plan could improve participation rates in resistance training programs.

The research is now clear that muscle strength is the new vital sign of the worker's physical health. Musculo-skeletal health of the worker can be improved. When a worker maintains good muscular strength, the worker is more productive and has fewer medical claims.

Conflict of interest

The authors declare no conflicts of interest with respect to research, authorship and/or publication of this article.

Author details

Thomas Gilliam[1*] and Paul Terpeluk[2]

1 IPCS, Hudson, OH, USA

2 Cleveland Clinic, Cleveland, OH, USA

*Address all correspondence to: tgilliam@ipcs-inc.com

References

[1] Wolfe RR. The underappreciated role of muscle in health and disease. Am J Clin Nutr. 2006;84:475-82.

[2] Carvalho CJD, Longo GZ, Kakehasi AM, Pereira PF, Segheto, KJ, Juvanhol, LL, Ribeiro, AQ. Association between skeletal mass indices and metabolic syndrome in Brazilian adults. J Clinical Densitometry. 2020. DOI: 10.1016/j.jocd.2020.02.003

[3] Kravitz LR. Developing a lifelong resistance training program. ACSM's Health & Fitness Journal. 2019;23(1):9-15

[4] Argiles JM, Campos N, Lopez-Pedrosa JM, Rueda R, Rodriquez-Manas L. Skeletal muscle regulates metabolism via interorgan crosstalk: roles in health and disease. JAMDA. 2016;17:789-796. DOI: 10.1016/j.jamda.2016.04.019

[5] Mrowka R. Westphal A. Skeletal muscle in the fight for chronic diseases. Acta Physiologica. 2018;223:e13086. DOI: 10.1111/alpha. 13086

[6] Mohamed AA, Alawna M. Role of increasing the aerobic capacity on improving the function of immune and respiratory systems in patients with coronavirus (COVID-19): A review. Diabetes & Metabolic Syndrome: Clinical Research & Reviews. 2020;14:489-496. DOI: 10.1016/j.dsx.2020.04.038.

[7] LaVoy ECP, Fagundes CP, Dantzer R. Exercise, inflammation, and fatigue in cancer survivors. Exerc Immunol Review. 2016;22:82-93.

[8] Simpson RJ, Campbell JP, Gleeson M, Kruger K, Nieman DC, Pyne DB, Turner JE, Walsh NP. Can exercise affect immune function to increase susceptibility to infection? Exerc Immunol Review. 2020;26:8-22.

[9] Nieman DC, Wentz LM. The compelling link between physical activity and the body's defense system. J Sport Health Sci. 2019;8:201-217. DOI: 10.1016/j.jshs.2018.09.009.

[10] Mesinovic J, Zengin A, DeCourten B, Ebling PR, Scott D. Sarcopenia and Type 2 diabetes mellitus: a bidirectional relationship. Diabetes, Metabolic Syndrome and Obesity: Targets and Therapy. 2019;12:1057-1072.

[11] Lu Y, Niti M, Yap KB, Tan CTY, Nyunt MSZ, Feng L, Tan BY, Chan G, Khoo SH, Chan SM, Yap P, Larbi A, Ng TP. Assessment of sarcopenia among community-dwelling at risk frail adults aged 65 years and older who received multidomain lifestyle interventions: A secondary analysis of a randomized clinical trial. JAMA Network Open. 2019;2(10):e1913346. DOI: 10.1001/jamanetworkopen.2019.13346.

[12] Machado KLLL. Domiciano DS, Machado LG, Lopes JB, Figueiredo CP, Caparbo VF, Takayama L, Menezes PR, Pereira RMR. Risk factors for low muscle mass in a population-based prospective chohort of Brazilian community-dwelling older women: The Sao Paulo Aging & Health (SPAH) Study. J Clinical Densitometry. 2019. DOI: 10.1016/j.jocd.2019.05.001.

[13] Manini TM, Clark BC. Dynapenia and aging: An update. J Gerontol A Biol Sci Med Sci. 2012;67A(1):28-40. DOI: 10.1093/Gerona/glr010

[14] Abdalla PP, dos Santos Carvalho A, dos Santos AP, Venturina ACR, Alves TC, Mota J, Machado DRL. One-repetition submaximal protocol to measure knee extensors muscle strength among older adults with and without sarcopenia: a validation study. BMC Sports Science, Medicine and Rehabilitation. 2020;12:29. DOI: 10.1186/s13102-020-00178-9.

[15] Thompson CJ, Holskey TH, Wallenrod S, Simunovich S, Corn R. Effectiveness of a fall prevention exercise program on falls risk in community-dwelling older adults. Translational Journal of the ACSM. 2019;4(3):16-22.

[16] Vlietstra, Hendrickx. Exercise interventions in healthy older adults with sarcopenia: A systematic review and meta-analysis. Australasian Journal on Aging. 2018;37(3):169-183. DOI: 10.1111/ajag.12521.

[17] Tomeleri CM, Ribeiro AS, Souza MF, Schiavoni D, Schoenfeld BJ, Venturini D, Barbosa DS, Landucci K, Sardinha LB, Cyrino ES. Resistance training improves inflammatory level, lipid and glycemic profiles in obese older women: A randomized controlled trial. Experimental Gerontology. 2016;84:80-87. DOI: 10.1016/j.exger.2016.09.005.

[18] Caan BJ, Feliciano EMS, Prado CM, Alexeeff S, Kroenke CH, Bradshaw P, QuesenberryCP,WeltzienEK,CastilloAL, Olobatuyi TA, Chen WY. Association of muscle and adiposity measured by computed tomography with survival in patients with nonmetastatic breast cancer. JAMA Oncology. 2018. DOI: 10.1001/jamaoncol.2018.0137.

[19] Feliciano EMC, Kroenke CH, Meyerhardt JA, Prado CM, Bradshw PT,Kwan ML, Xiao J, Alexeff S, Corley C, Weltzien E, Castillo AL, Caan BJ. Association of systemic inflammation and sarcopenia with survival in nonmetastatic colorectal cancer: Results from the C SCANS study. JAMA Oncol. 2017;3(12):e172319. DOI: 10.1001/jamaoncol.2017.2319.

[20] Williams GR, Chen Y, Kenzik KM, McDonald A, Shachaar SS, Klepiin HD Kritchevsky S, Bhatia S. Assessment of sarcopenia measures, survival, and disability in older adults before and after diagnosis with cancer. JAMA Network Open. 2020;3(5):e204783. DOI: 10.1001/jamanetworkopen.2020.4783.

[21] Gilchrist SC, Howard VJ, Akinyemiju T, Judd SE, Cushman M, Hooker SP, Diaz KM. Association of sedentary behavior with cancer mortality in middle-aged and older US adults. JAMA Oncology. 2020;6(8):1210-1217. DOI:10.1001/jamaoncol.2020.2045.

[22] Brown JM, Shackelford DYK, Hipp ML, Hayward R. Evaluation of an exercise-based phase program as part of a standard care model for cancer survivors. Translational Journal of the ACSM. 2019;4(7):45-54.

[23] Campbell KL, Winters-Stone KM, Wiskemann J, May AM, Schwartz AL, Courneya KS, Zucker DS, Matthews CE, Ligibel JA, Gerber LH, Morris GS, Patel AV, H TF, Perna FM Schmitz KH. Exercise guidelines for cancer survivors: Consensus statement for international multidisciplinary roundtable. Medicine & Science in Sports Medicine. 2019;51(11):2375-2390. DOI: 10.1249/MSS.0000000000002116.

[24] Cheema BS, Fairman CM, Marthick M. Exercise professionals in the cancer center: Experiences, recommendations, and future research. Translational Journal of ACSM. 2019;4(1):96-105.

[25] Schmitz KH, Campbell AM, Stuiver MM, Pinto BM, Swhwartz AL, Morris GS, Ligibel JA, Cheville A, Galvao DA, Alfno CM, Patel AV, Hue T, Gerber LH, Sallis, R, Gusani NJ, Stout NL, Chan L, Flowers F, Doyle C, Hemmrich S, Bain W, Sokolof J, WintersStone, KM, Campbell KL, Matthews CE. Exercise is medicine in oncology: Engaging clinicians to help patients move through cancer. CA Cancer J Clin. 2019;0:1-17.

[26] Patel AV, Friedenreich CM, Moore SC, Hayes SC, Silver JK, Campbell KL, Winters-stone K, Gerber LH, George SM, Fulton JE,

Denlinger C, Morris GS, Hue T, Schmitz KH, Matthews CE. American College of Sports Medicine roundtable report on physical activity, sedentary behavior, and cancer prevention and control. Med Sci Sports Exerc. 2019;51(11):2391-2402. DOI: 10.1249/MSS0000000000002117.

[27] Mctiernan A, Friedenreich CM, Katzmarzyk PT, Powell KE, Macko R, Buchner D, Pescatello LS, Bloodgood B, Tennant B, Vaux-Bjerke A, George SM, Troiano RP, Piercy KL. Physical activity in cancer prevention and survival: A systemic review. Med Sci Sports Exerc. 2019;51(6):1252-1261. DOI: 10.1249/MSS.0000000000001937.

[28] Haran PA, Rivas DA. Role and potential mechanisms of anabolic resistance in sarcopenia. J Cachexia Sarcopenia Muscle. 2012;3:157-162. DOI: 10.1007/s13539-012-0068-4.

[29] Garcia-HermosoA,Cavero-RedondoI, Ramirez-Valez R, Ruiz JR, Ortega FB, Lee DC, Martinez-Vizcaino V. Muscular strength as a predictor of all-cause mortality in an apparently healthy population: A systematic review and meta-analysis of data from approximately 2 million men and women. Archives of Physical Medicine and Rehabilitation. 2018;99:2100-2113. DOI: 10.1016/j.apmr.2018.01.008.

[30] Moberg M, Lindholm ME, Reitzner SM, Ekblom B, Sundberg CJ, Psilander N. Exercise induces different molecular responses in trained and untrained human muscle. Med Sci Sports Exerc. 2020;52(8):1679-1690. DOI: 10.1249/MSS.0000000000002310.

[31] Abramowitz MK, Hall CB, Amodu A, Sharma D, Androga L, Hawkins M. Muscle mass, BMI, and mortality among adults in the United States: A population-based cohort study. PLOS One. 2018. DOI: 10.1371/journal.pone.0194697.

[32] Churchward-Venne TA, Tieland M, Verdijk LB, Leenders M, Dirks ML, DeGroot LCPGM. There are no nonresponders to resistance-type exercise training in older men and women. JAMDA. 2015;16:400-411. DOI: 10.1016/j.jamda.2015.01.071.

[33] Dai X, Zhai L, Chen Q, Miller JD, Lu L, Hsue C, Lie L, Yuan X, Wei W, Ma X, Fang Z, Zhao W, Lie Y, Huang F, Lou Q. Two-year-supervised resistance training prevented diabetes incidence in people with prediabetes: A randomized control trial. Diabetes Metab Res Rev. 2019;35:e3143. DOI: 10.1002/dmmr.3143.

[34] Beaumont C, Ferrara PMM, Strohacker K. Measurements of acute affective responses to resistance training exercise: A narrative review. Translational Journal of the ACSM. 2020;5(11):1-7.

[35] Church TS, Thomas DM, Tudor-Locke C, Katzmarzyk PT, Earnest CP, Rodarte RQ, Martin CK, Blair SN, Bouchard C. Trends over 5 decades in U.S. occupation-related physical activity and their associations with obesity. PLOS One. 2011;6(5):e19657. DOI. 10.1371/journal.pone.0019657.

[36] Brighenti-Zoag S, Mundwiler J, Schupbach U, Dieterie T, Wolfer DP, Leuppi JD, Miedinger D. Physical workload and work capacity across occupational groups. PLOS One. 2016. DOI: 10.1371/journal.pone.0154073.

[37] Industrial Physical Capability Services, Inc. (IPCS). Available from http://www.ipcs-inc.com.

[38] Biodex. 2020. Biodex System 4 Pro™ [Apparatus and software]. Available from http://www.biodex/physical-medicine/products/dynamometers/system-4-pro.

[39] Ostbye T, Dement JM, Krause KM. Obesity and workers compensation. Arch Intern Med. 2007;167:766-773.

[40] Terpeluk P, Rogen B, Gilliam T. Medical and pharmacy costs for new hire nurses following a physical strength evaluation screening in a large health system. Workplace Health & Safety. 2016;64(9):420-425. DOI: 10.1177/2165079915621317.

[41] Dictionary of Occupational Titles Appendix C: Components of the definition trailer. 2015. Retrieved from http://www.lb7.uscourts.gov/documents/11c2448.pdf.

Chapter 8

Physiological Stress Responses Associated with High-Risk Occupational Duties

Jennifer F. Chan and Judith P. Andersen

Abstract

Occupational stress is a pervasive problem that is relevant across the world. Stress, in combination with occupational hazards, may pose additive risks for health and wellbeing. This chapter discusses the influence of physical and psychosocial stressors on basal cortisol regulation as associated with higher-risk occupational duties among two subspecialties of police officers (frontline and special tactical unit officers). Results reveal significant differences in dysregulated cortisol awakening response associated with the higher risk duties among special tactical unit officers. In contrast, frontline officers with a lower objective occupational risk profiles report higher subjective stress levels. Dysregulated or maladaptive cortisol levels are associated with increased health risk. Thus, individuals working in high stress occupations with elevated cortisol profiles may be at increased risk of chronic health conditions. Results suggest that considering both objective physiological markers and subjective reports of stress are dually important aspects in designing interventions for police officers of differing subspecialties.

Keywords: stress, diurnal cortisol, occupational risk, HPA, fight-or-flight, police

1. Introduction

Most of the world's population spends approximately a third of their adult life at work [1]. Interestingly, work also consistently remains a top cited source of adult stress (64% of 3602 surveyed United States adults) [2]. In the context of occupational health, the World Health Organization (WHO) defines occupational stress as the response when presented with work demands that do not match knowledge and abilities, thus, challenging the individual's ability to cope; research suggests the most stressful types of work are those that provide excessive demands and pressures, low perception of control, and provides little support from others [3]. Occupational stress can manifest in physical symptoms, especially cardiovascular ailments; stress is linked to seven of the top ten causes of death in the world, with heart disease being the leading cause for men and women, and chronic occupational stress increasing coronary heart disease risk by 40–50% [4–6].

With occupational stress cited as such a pervasive part of our lives, there is great interest to better understand the impact that stress, in combination with objective occupational hazards, may have on physical and mental health. Thus it is critical to better understand how different workplace factors contribute to or exacerbate stress. As occupational duties and stress exposure varies across occupations, occupational stress sources (i.e., stressors) can be further separated into operational stressors (i.e., job content-inherent aspects of the occupation) and organizational stressors (i.e., job context-characteristics and behaviors of the organization and people of them) [7]. One route to understand how different levels of occupational stress can affect the body is by looking to varying levels of occupational risk exposure within a single occupation via its operational stressors.

Researchers have specialized in examining the effects of occupational responsibilities [7–9], comparing risk subtypes within a high-risk occupation [10]. In a previous study [10], the authors focused on identifying the objective physiological stress associated with risk-subtype among police officers in comparison to the general public. This prior literature revealed that police had significantly higher physiological stress responses (i.e., basal cortisol regulation) in comparison to the general population, with the effect even more pronounced as objective occupational hazards increased (i.e., frontline vs. tactical police).

The goal of this chapter is to discuss stress of varying occupational risk profiles and objective hazards' impact on physiological stress response, while considering participants' subjective reports of stress. Specifically, the authors present analyses to assess subjective measures of stress to further stratify and identify specific factors that may drive objective physiological stress (i.e., basal cortisol regulation) trends observed in a police sample. We hypothesized a positive association between increased risk associated with objective occupational hazards and self-reported stressors. Specifically, that dysregulation in HPA function would be higher among tactical unit officers and this would align with both increased occupational hazards (objective) and self-reported occupational stressors (subjective).

2. The "fight-or-flight" response

Evolutionarily speaking, stress and our ability to respond to it is adaptive and essential for our survival. When presented with a potential threat, the body automatically engages in a series of adaptive physiological processes to maximize survival [11]. Colloquially this process is known as the "fight-or-flight" response. During fight-or-flight, the autonomic nervous system's (ANS) two sub-systems are engaged: the sympathetic nervous system (SNS) is activated, and the parasympathetic nervous system (PNS—responsible for calming and stabilizing the body) is suppressed. The Hypothalamic–Pituitary–Adrenal (HPA) axis is a critical system, producing a cascade of hormones that both maintain and dampen the fight-or-flight response when a threat is presented or removed, respectively.

While fight-or-flight is strictly a physiological response, it can be maintained and stimulated by psychological processes. The degree of activation among the SNS, PNS, and HPA axis is determined by an individual's perception of how threatening the stimulus is, and can be influenced by psychological factors (e.g., threat perception, anxiety, anticipation, perceived control over the situation, etc.) [12]. When a stimulus is perceived as stressful, the hypothalamus releases corticotropin-releasing hormone (CRH), which subsequently triggers the pituitary gland to release of adrenocorticotropic hormone (ACTH). ACTH travels in the bloodstream to the adrenal glands, located above the kidneys, triggering the release of stress hormones glucocorticoids (i.e., cortisol) and catecholamines (e.g., epinephrine, and norepinephrine) [13].

Stress hormones act upon the SNS and PNS, and higher priority survival functions such as heart rate, respiration, energy reserves, and short-term immunity are increased, while lower priority functions for threat response such as reproduction, gastrointestinal activity, and long-term immunity are suppressed [14]. As a result, prolonged dysregulation of HPA activity can have systemic negative effects on regulatory processes in the body, thus increasing the risk of health conditions.

2.1 Cortisol

Cortisol (i.e., glucocorticoids) is a key regulating stress hormone in the human HPA axis cascade. Cortisol potentiates the effects of catecholamines on beta receptors (necessary for impacting peripheral receptors), suppresses immune function, and terminates the fight-or-flight response (via negative feedback loop) [15]. Cortisol is excreted in a dose–response manner to the level of perceived threat by the individual, meaning the greater the perceived threat, the more cortisol that is excreted [16].

Cortisol also has important regulatory functions outside times of stress; cortisol is additionally excreted in a systemic diurnal pattern over every 24-hour period cycle. Among healthy individuals, the diurnal pattern consists of higher levels upon waking, a significant peak around 30 minutes post-waking (i.e., the cortisol awakening response—CAR), steady decline throughout the day, and reaches its lowest point in the middle of the night before again elevating again in the early hours of the next day [17].

2.2 Health risks of maladaptive stress responses

A normal diurnal cortisol pattern indicates individual ability to maintain and return to homeostasis after experiencing stress [16, 18, 19]. However, chronic or repeated stress and subsequent over-activation of the fight-or-flight response can exhaust the HPA axis, resulting in excessive cortisol secretion and eventually, dysregulated diurnal cortisol cycles. Systemically, cortisol influences a wide range of organs and functions including blood pressure regulation and metabolic activity [13, 20]. Thus, long-term, dysregulated cortisol levels significantly increase potential physical and mental illness risks [21]. Physical issues include but are not limited to, compromised immunity, diabetes, hypertension, and cardiovascular disease. Mental health associations include development of depression, anxiety, and psychophysiological PTSD symptoms, such as hyperarousal, and elevated heart rate [22, 23]. Measuring diurnal cortisol patterns, and distinguishing maladaptive patterns and their associated triggers, are critical for identifying potential health risks in populations.

3. High-risk occupations

High-risk occupations present a useful framework for studying the effect of chronic stress on health. By definition, high-risk occupations include work that may be disproportionately exposed to hazardous work environments (e.g., construction, materials handling, emergency response, military) [24]. High-risk occupations imply greater exposure to situations considered potentially dangerous, harmful, or threatening, and potentially, chronically elevated stress responses and excessive cortisol release. Studying the effects of stress in high-risk occupations is also important when taking into consideration performance and duties that are expected to be executed when under stress. Occupational stress that influences performance can result in errors, lower productivity, burnout, or workplace injury, affecting not only the individual but straining the infrastructure of their workplace and health resources [25]. While there are many different types of high-risk occupations, this chapter will focus on the occupation of policing and two subspecialties as an example, given the authors' existing expertise in first responder stress, both from a physiological and psychological standpoint.

3.1 Police stress

Police are often the first to arrive to emergencies where they are regularly exposed to dangerous or threatening situations which pose possible harm to their physical and mental health. Previous literature has established that police exhibit stress responses during active duty and in training [26, 27]. Police occupational stress is significantly linked to poorer health, including lower physical and mental health, and higher physician-diagnosed morbidity, cardiovascular disease, and metabolic syndrome [28]. Heightened anticipatory threat anxiety in these high pressure environments can also result in reduced attentional control that influences active performance [29] and decision making tasks [30] (e.g., motor execution, inhibitory control, use-of-force decisions). Because police health significantly impacts their performance and communities, researchers have focused on understanding how models of physiological stress may apply to their operational stress conditions.

While previous research on police diurnal cortisol focused on the effects of factors such as shift-work, posttraumatic stress disorder (PTSD), sleep quality, and cardiovascular disease, there was limited research providing baseline norms for diurnal cortisol patterns as a function of occupational risk. Our research group has addressed an existing gap in the literature by examining diurnal cortisol patterns of police officers from different risk subspecialties, specifically, frontline and tactical police [10]. Frontline police officers' duties include direct interaction with members of the community in response to unlawful acts witnessed while on patrol, or civilian-reported events. As frontline officers are frequently first to arrive to the scene, they also determine if further specialty units are needed to resolve an incident. Specialty units within a police service, such as tactical teams, are equipped with skills, tools, and training to respond to the highest risk incidents that are beyond the capabilities of an average frontline officer (e.g., active shooter events, barricaded suspects, hostage situations); in many police organizations, tactical units are required to first serve as a frontline officer before enrolling in specialized training to obtain and maintain advanced skills for such incidents [31, 32].

The authors' prior work revealed objective evidence that police had higher diurnal cortisol patterns in comparison to the general population, especially within 30 minutes of waking (CAR). Cortisol levels also differed in respect to police subspecialties. Specifically, tactical officers (the highest risk subspecialty) displayed significantly higher CAR in comparison to frontline officers.

3.2 Present study

The goal of the present chapter is to take a deeper dive and stratify physiological differences between risk-subspecialties, by focusing on officers' subjective reported stress. Because tactical officers have higher objective physiological stress and risk exposure, we expect that tactical police will report higher levels of subjective stress in comparison to frontline police.

3.2.1 Participants

Frontline Officers (n = 57, 14% female) consisted of police constable level volunteers from a Canadian municipal police force (M_{Age} = 32.80, SD = 6.29;

M_{Exp} = 7.09 years, SD = 5.63). Of the 57 participants, 52 provided complete cortisol samples, and 55 provided complete survey data. Inclusion criteria required frontline officers who completed the entirety of their training, and deemed healthy and fit for active duty (as per standards defined and measured by their police service). Exclusion criteria included non-frontline law enforcement or civilian workers, and officers on leave or deemed unfit for duty.

Tactical Officers (n = 44, all male; M_{Age} = 32.31, SD = 3.79; M_{Exp} = 4.66 years, SD = 3.98) were comprised of three active duty Finnish Special Response Teams: two regional-level (n = 32, M_{Age} = 32.14, SD = 4.26) and one federal-level (n = 12, M_{Age} = 31.50, SD = 2.02) the tactical teams were tested within 6 months of one another. All tactical officers provided complete cortisol and survey data. Inclusion criteria allowed for any tactical team members deemed fit or healthy by their police agency. Exclusion criteria included non-tactical officers or civilian workers, and officers deemed unfit for duty.

3.2.2 Cortisol collection and measurement

For full details of cortisol collection and measurement, refer to Planche et al. [10]. Police participants were instructed to use the passive drool method to collect saliva samples into a collection tube at four time points: immediately upon waking, 30 minutes following wake, before dinner (11 hours post waking), and before bed (~17 hours post waking). Participants were instructed they should not eat, drink, or brush their teeth within the hour before the sample collection. After collection, samples were frozen for preservation until analyses.

Frontline officers' cortisol levels were determined with enzyme-linked immunosorbent assay (ELISA) kits (No. 80957; Crystal Chem, Elk Grove Village, Illinois), using a plate reader (Biotek, Winooski, Vermont) and commercial software (Gen 5) to quantify cortisol concentration.

Tactical officers' cortisol samples were collected in Finland and were shipped to an independent laboratory for analyses (Clemens Kirschbaum, Technische Universitat Dresden, DE). Salivary cortisol concentrations were measured using commercially available chemiluminescence-immuno-assay with high sensitivity (IBL assay; IBL International, Hamburg, Germany).

To compare frontline and tactical police cortisol levels to the general population, data were extrapolated from **Figure 1** of Miller et al., 2016's North American and European meta-dataset of diurnal salivary cortisol [33]. Salivary cortisol levels were restricted to studies using the Delfia-assay (Dressendörfer et al., 1992, University of Trier) or the IBL chemiluminescence-assay depending on the field study. Average diurnal cortisol value for each of the 10th, 25th, 50th, and 75th, and 90th percentiles general population (15 studies, n = 18,698) for the same time points collected in the frontline and tactical police samples (wake, 30 minutes post-wake, 11 hours post-wake, and 17 hours post-wake).

3.2.3 Subjective stress

Subjective stress was measured via the Police Stress Questionnaire (PSQ). The PSQ is a 40-item self-report questionnaire that measures police stress across two subscales (organizational stressors—20 questions, operational stressors—20 questions). Participants are asked to rate stress for each item on a 7-point Likert scale ("No stress" (1) – "Moderate stress" (4) – "A lot of stress" (7)) experienced over the prior 6 months. The PSQ displays high internal consistency on both subscales (Cronbach's α = 0.93Op, 0.92Org); it also has good construct, discriminant, and convergent validity, with low shared variance between the subscales, low shared variance to other general stress measures, and positively correlates with other measures of job satisfaction [34]. For this study, the 20 items of the operational stress subscale of the PSQ (PSQ-Op) was used for measuring self-reported subjective operational job-context related stress in frontline and tactical police officers.

3.2.4 Data analysis

Pairwise comparisons confirmed that tactical regional and federal-level subsamples did not significantly differ from each other across all time points for cortisol and self-reported stress data, and sufficient to combine regional and federal subsamples into a single tactical sample group.

For subjective stress comparisons, self-reported stress responses on the PSQ had a non-normal distribution violating the assumptions of a t-test. Therefore, a Wilcoxon rank sum test was used to compare overall reported stress between frontline and tactical officers.

Average diurnal cortisol levels were calculated for each police participant at each time point. Factorial ANOVA was performed to compare specific diurnal time point cortisol levels across each group. Repeated-measures mixed-model analysis of variance (ANOVA) with Bonferroni corrections was used to compare multiple pairwise differences in cortisol levels between groups across time points.

3.2.5 Objective physiological police stress results

As previously cited in Planche et al. [10], ANOVA comparisons for between-group diurnal cortisol differences revealed that police officers had significantly higher levels of cortisol at all collected time points in comparison to the general population ($p < 0.05$). In comparison to frontline officers, tactical officers displayed significantly higher levels of cortisol at awakening and 30 minutes post-awakening in comparison to the frontline officers ($p < 0.05$), non-significantly different levels 11-hours post ($p > 0.05$), and significantly lower levels of cortisol at 17 h post ($p < 0.05$) (See **Figure 1**).

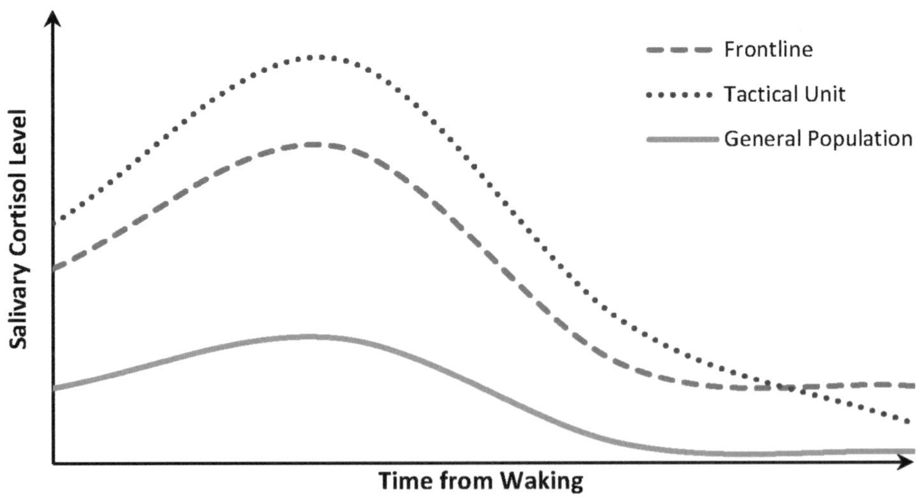

Figure 1.
Overview of diurnal salivary cortisol relationships across 17 h from waking in frontline police (n = 52), tactical police (n = 44), and the general population (n = 18,698). Adapted from Planche et al., 2019.

3.2.6 Subjective police stress results

Using Wilcoxon rank sum testing, frontline officers self-reported significantly higher total levels of operational stress in comparison to tactical officers ($Median_{Frontline} = 56$, IQR = 33; $Median_{Tactical} = 44$, IQR = 16; $p < 0.05$) with small effect (r = 0.26) (See **Figure 2**).

When comparing the means across PSQ-Op items (See **Table 1**), the two groups had the largest magnitude differences (ΔMean), with frontline reporting greater stress, on: negative comments from the public, upholding a "higher image" in public, over-time demands, and lack of understanding from family and friends about work. Furthermore, these four items fell within the six lowest reported sources of operational stress for tactical officers. In comparison, tactical officers reported more objective risk items such as being injured on the job, traumatic events, and working alone at night as higher levels of stress in comparison to frontline. For both groups, fatigue, paperwork, and not enough time available to spend with family were ranked among the highest sources of stress.

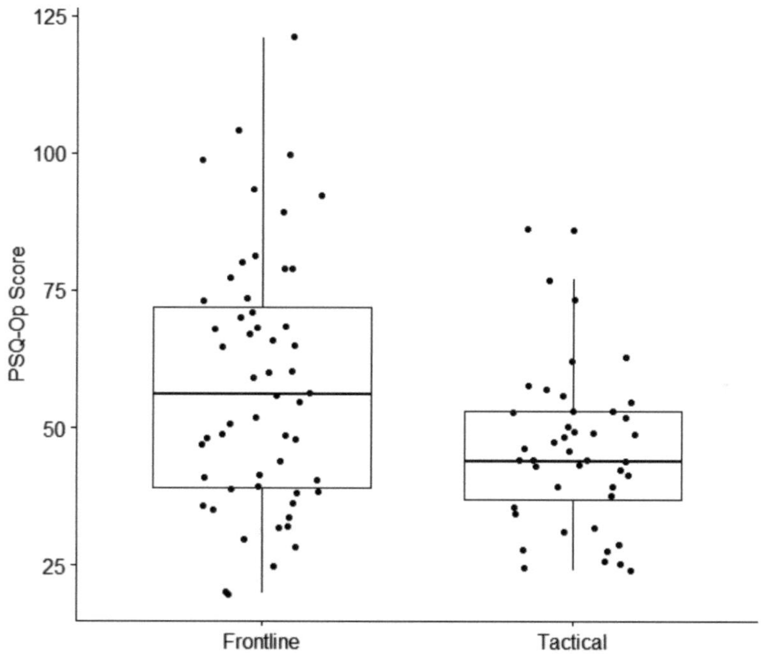

Figure 2.
Boxplot distribution of police (frontline and tactical) total scores on the PSQ-Op. Frontline officers self-reported significantly higher total levels of operational stress in comparison to tactical officers (p < 0.05).

3.3 Discussion

The aim of the current study was to discern potential differences of tactical and frontline police officers' subjective self-reported stress, and the relationship to objective occupational hazard profiles. It was expected that, similar to previous findings of police objective stress (i.e., diurnal salivary cortisol), officers from tactical teams would report significantly higher levels of subjective stress on the PSQ-Op in comparison to frontline officers. However, in contrast to our hypotheses, Wilcoxon rank sum testing revealed that 1) frontline officers reported significantly

PSQ-Op Item	Frontline mean(SD)	Tactical mean(SD)	ΔMean
Total Police Operational Stress Score	**57.95(23.08)**	**45.60(13.90)**	**12.35**
Shift work	3.20(1.64)	3.16(1.27)	0.04
Working alone at night	2.28(1.32)	2.15(1.20)	0.13
Over-time demands	2.91(1.69)	1.69(0.84)	1.22
Risk of being injured on the job	2.53(1.68)	2.47(1.08)	0.06
Work related activities on days off (e.g. court, community events)	3.00(1.59)	2.65(1.62)	0.35
Traumatic events (e.g. MVA, domestics, death, injury)	2.56(1.49)	2.26(1.24)	0.30
Managing your social life outside of work	2.89(1.65)	2.47(1.24)	0.42
Not enough time available to spend with friends and family	3.25(1.67)	2.88(1.53)	0.37
Paperwork	3.51(2.03)	2.84(1.33)	0.67
Eating healthy at work	3.11(1.69)	2.30(1.01)	0.81
Finding time to stay in good physical condition	3.40(1.62)	2.65(1.31)	0.75
Fatigue (e.g. shift work, over-time)	3.65(1.79)	3.28(1.50)	0.37
Occupation-related health issues (e.g. back pain)	3.02(1.69)	2.26(1.20)	0.76
Lack of understanding from family and friends about your work	2.70(1.69)	1.67(0.64)	1.03
Making friends outside the job	2.24(1.53)	1.84(1.00)	0.40
Upholding a "higher image" in public	3.00(1.72)	1.58(0.66)	1.42
Negative comments from the public	3.40(1.98)	1.86(1.01)	1.54
Limitations to your social life (e.g. who your friends are, where you socialize)	2.72(1.52)	1.74(0.98)	0.98
Feeling like you are always on the job	2.73(1.72)	2.14(1.28)	0.59
Friends / family feel the effects of the stigma associated with your job	2.31(1.40)	2.02(1.18)	0.29

Table 1.
Frontline (n = 55) and tactical police (n = 44) mean and standard deviation (SD) scores for total PSQ-Op sum, as well as individual items, and magnitude difference scores between frontline and tactical (ΔMean). Average stress level of each item compared to recommended PSQ-Op cut-off scores: Low stress (≤2.0), moderate stress (2.1–3.4), high stress (≥3.5) [34].

higher levels of overall subjective stress in comparison to tactical officers, and 2) frontline and tactical police reported qualitatively different stressors, with tactical police reporting more work-related objective stressors, and frontline police reporting more public-image related stressors.

Results are discussed within the limitations of the study. First, due to the difficulty of recruiting police samples, this study consisted of smaller sample sizes, which limits its generalization capabilities. Second, this is data is strictly correlational, thus causal relationships cannot be stated. However, we can review the data results within the lens of modern policing in regards to the following perspectives:

1. The current media spotlight focused on frontline officers, including psychological expectations and demands

2. Physical fitness requirements of tactical versus frontline police

3.3.1 Stress and psychological demands

While the subjective stress findings countered our hypothesis, they may be explained by current issues and pressures in modern policing. Rising issues and media coverage of police incidents such as excessive use of force, systemic racism, and criminal charges, continue to erode the public's trust, as well as damage the police-community relationship [35, 36]. This inference is further bolstered by the findings of this study that frontline officers considered PSQ-Op items related to public image greater of sources of stress than tactical officers did. In comparison, tactical officers are only called to the most high-risk and violent situations (e.g., hostage, school shootings, etc.) and in comparison to frontline police are less in the spotlight, thus aligning with the current study results that subjective stress reported by tactical officers reflected primarily objective operational stressors (i.e., risk to life).

Due to the duties of a tactical officer, they are much more likely to encounter life-threatening situations. CAR can also represent psychological anticipation of the day, with higher demands predicting a more pronounced CAR [37]. Given officers' pre-existing awareness of the increased risk associated with joining a tactical unit, individuals with certain personality characteristics or physiological profiles (e.g., cortisol) may be self-selecting towards higher-risk occupational roles. However, this theory is difficult to test without longitudinal data about individuals prior to entering a high-risk occupation of any kind.

3.3.2 Stress and physical demands

Another possible explanation as to why the results reveal a higher objective stress profile but lower subjective stress profile among tactical officers compared to frontline may be due to the physical condition of tactical officers in comparison to frontline officers. By demand of their duties, tactical teams are required to remain in good health and take part in many hours of specialized training, including physical fitness [38–40]. Higher levels of exercise have been found to affect diurnal cortisol patterns, particularly CAR, in lower-risk occupations, the general population, and athletes. Increased regular exercise has been shown to increase CAR; seniors who completed a 6-month aerobic exercise intervention displayed significant increased CAR, but not associated with changes in diurnal cortisol as measured by area under the curve (AUC) [41]. Similarly, high-performance athletes also exhibit higher diurnal cortisol patterns including an elevated CAR response [42]. These findings parallel the results of the present study, in which tactical teams display elevated CAR, but maintain similar cortisol levels to frontline officers later in the day.

By the same token, evidence suggests that frontline officers do not meet the same level of physical fitness requirements as tactical officers. Frontline officers in this study were not required to maintain physical fitness, rather it remained the responsibility of the individual officer [43, 44]. With further support from findings of the present study, frontline officers reported finding time to stay in good physical condition as a higher source of stress on the PSQ-Op than tactical officers did, suggesting frontline officers have greater difficulty maintaining exercise as part of daily routine. Due to the original design of the study, it is difficult to determine whether the physiological and subjective stress differences between tactical and frontline are exercise related. However, future research could control for exercise by targeting frontline and tactical samples with the same exercise regiments and practices and compare their cortisol levels to rule out this possibility.

3.3.3 Implications

Within the limitations of the current study, results suggest that both frontline and tactical officers display dysregulated cortisol patterns that are associated with their higher-risk occupational duties in comparison to the general population (see also [10]). This places officers at higher risk of negative health outcomes (e.g., greater rates of mental illness and cardiovascular disease) [21, 45]. Furthermore, the subjective stress reported by officers differs by subspecialty and may inform intervention strategies aimed at mitigating officer stress and assisting with the regulation physiological stress, specifically CAR profiles.

Of note, the top rated operational stressors for both frontline and tactical groups were fatigue, paperwork, and not enough time available to spend with family. These subjective factors may significantly drive the elevated diurnal cortisol patterns across the entire day observed in comparison to the general population. If this relationship is true, these same stressors are often found or can be applied to a vast number of occupations, and it can be inferred that the presence of these stressors would potentially have the similar impact and associated health risks for other occupational groups.

4. Conclusion

While the stress response is beneficial from an evolutionary standpoint, chronic activation associated with occupational duties results in an excessive CAR profile, placing the worker at higher risk for negative health outcomes. High-risk occupations provide a framework for analyzing the effect of different stress exposure on physiology. While previous research has found that different risk- subspecialties of policing display increased cortisol patterns in line with increasing risk, follow-up analyses of subjective stress measures of the same groups found an opposite relationship, with lower-risk subtypes reporting higher levels of operational stress despite lower CAR profiles. Differentiating relationships provided an opportunity to explore the nuances of occupational stress profiles, and explanations of several other factors that also have impact (e.g., exercise and public image concerns). Results may inform tailored interventions to reduce both objective, physiological stress profiles (i.e., CAR response) and subjective self-reported stress profiles among high-risk occupational subspecialties.

Acknowledgements

The authors would like to acknowledge and thank the Health Adaptation Research on Trauma (HART) Lab research assistants and volunteers in who assisted in the data collection, coding, and cleaning. Thank you to the agency who collaborated with us to make the data collection possible, and to all the police officers who participated in the study.

Conflict of interest

The authors declare no conflict of interest.

Author details

Jennifer F. Chan and Judith P. Andersen*
University of Toronto Mississauga, Mississauga, Canada

*Address all correspondence to: judith.andersen@utoronto.ca

References

[1] World Health Organization. Global strategy on occupational health for all: The way to health at work [Internet]. 1994. Available from: https://www.who.int/occupational_health/publications/globstrategy/en/index2.html [Accessed: 2020-08-25]

[2] American Psychological Association. Stress in America™ 2019 [Internet]. 1994. Available from: https://www.apa.org/news/press/releases/stress/2019/stress-america-2019.pdf [Accessed: 2020-08-25]

[3] World Health Organization. Stress at the workplace [Internet]. n.d. Available from: https://www.who.int/occupational_health/topics/stressatwp/en/ [Accessed: 2020-08-25]

[4] Quick, JC, & Henderson, DF. Occupational stress: Preventing suffering, enhancing wellbeing. International Journal of Environmental Research and Public Health, 2016;13(5): 459. DOI: 10.3390/ijerph13050459

[5] World Health Organization. The top 10 causes of death [Internet]. 2018. Available from: https://www.who.int/news-room/fact-sheets/detail/the-top-10-causes-of-death [Accessed: 2020-08-25]

[6] Steptoe A, Kivimäki M. Stress and cardiovascular disease. Nature Reviews Cardiology 2012;9:360-370. DOI: 10.1038/nrcardio.2012.45

[7] Shane JM. Organizational stressors and police performance. Journal of Criminal Justice. 2010;38:807-818. DOI: 10.1016/j.jcrimjus.2010.05.008

[8] Chan JF, Andersen JP. Challenges of Cross-Sectional Survey Measures for Assessing Occupational and Organizational Stress Effects on Mental Health Among Police Officers. SAGE Publications Ltd; 2020. DOI: 10.4135/9781529740448

[9] Houdmont J, Kerr R, Randall R. Organisational psychosocial hazard exposures in UK policing: Management standards indicator tool reference values. Policing. 2012;35(1):182-197. DOI: 10.1108/13639511211215522

[10] Planche K, Chan JF, Di Nota PM, Beston B, Boychuk E, Collins PI, Andersen JP. Diurnal Cortisol Variation According to High-Risk Occupational Specialty Within Police: Comparisons Between Frontline, Tactical Officers, and the General Population. Journal of Occupational and Environmental Medicine. 2019;61(6):e260–e265. DOI: 10.1097/JOM.0000000000001591

[11] Thayer JF, Sternberg E. Beyond heart rate variability: Vagal regulation of allostatic systems. In Annals of the New York Academy of Sciences. 2006; 1088(1):361-372. DOI: 10.1196/annals.1366.014

[12] Kalish R, Müller MB, Tüscher O. A conceptual framework for the neurobiological study of resilience. Behavioural and Brain Sciences. 2015;38:1-79. DOI: 10.1017/S0140525X1400082X

[13] Lupien SJ. How to Measure Stress in Humans. Centre for Studies on Human Stress. 2013.

[14] McEwen BS, Lasley EN. The End of Stress as we Know It. 2nd ed. New York: Dana Press; 2002.

[15] Huether SE, McCance KL. Understanding pathophysiology. 5th ed. St. Louis: Elsevier; 2012. p. 440.

[16] Lovallo WR. Stress and Health: Biological and Psychological Interactions. 3rd ed. Thousand Oaks: Sage Publications, Inc.; 2016.

[17] Hellhammer DH, Wust S, Kudielka BM. Salivary cortisol as a biomarker in stress research. Psychoneuroendocrinology. 2009; 34(2): 163-171. DOI: 10.1016/j.psyneuen.2008.10.026

[18] Fries E, Dettenborn L, Kirschbaum C. The cortisol awakening response (CAR): facts and future directions. International Journal of Psychophysiology. 2009;72(1):67-73. DOI: 10.1016/j.ijpsycho.2008.03.014

[19] Clow A, Thorn L, Evans P, Hucklebridge F. The awakening cortisol response: methodological issues and significance. Stress. 2004;7(1):29-37. DOI:10.1080/10253890410001667205

[20] Arnaldi G, Scandali VM, Trementino L, Cardinaletti M, Appolloni G, Boscaro M. Pathophysiology of Dyslipidemia in Cushing's Syndrome. Neuroendocrinology. 2010;92:86-90. DOI: 10.1159/000314213

[21] Violanti JM, Andrew ME, Burchfiel CM, Dorn J, Hartley T, Miller DB. Posttraumatic Stress Symptoms and Subclinical Cardiovascular Disease in Police Officers. International Journal of Stress Management Psychological Association. 2006;13(4):541-554. DOI: 10.1037/1072-5245.13.4.541

[22] Rodrigues SM, LeDoux JE, Sapolsky RM. The influence of stress hormones on fear circuitry. Annual Review of Neuroscience. 2009;32:289-313. DOI: 10.1146/annurev.neuro.051508.135620

[23] Menning H, Renz A, Seifert J, Maercker A. Reduced mismatch negativity in posttraumatic stress disorder: A compensatory mechanism for chronic hyperarousal? International Journal of Psychophysiology. 2008;68(1):27-34. DOI: 10.1016/j.ijpsycho.2007.12.003

[24] World Health Organization. High-Risk Jobs and High-Risk Populations [Internet]. 2011. Available from: https://www.apa.org/wsh/past/2011/high-risk-jobs [Accessed: 2020-08-25]

[25] Gershon RR, Barocas B, Canton AN, Li X, Vlahov D. Mental, physical, and behavioral outcomes associated with perceived work stress in police officers. Criminal Justice and Behavior. 2009;36(3):275-289. DOI: 10.1177/0093854808330015

[26] Andersen JP, Pitel M, Weerasinghe A, Papazoglou K. Highly Realistic Scenario Based Training Simulates the Psychophysiology of Real World Use of Force Encounters: Implications for Improved Police Officer Performance. Journal of Law Enforcement. 2016;5(4):1-13. Retrieved from http://search.ebscohost.com/login.aspx?direct=true&db=i3h&AN=114681849&site=ehost-live

[27] Baldwin S, Bennell C, Andersen JP, Semple T, Jenkins B. Stress-Activity Mapping: Physiological Responses During General Duty Police Encounters. Frontiers in Psychology. 2019;10. DOI: 10.3389/fpsyg.2019.02216

[28] Violanti JM, Charles LE, McCanlies E, Hartley TA, Baughman P, Andrew ME, Fekedulegn D, Ma CC, Mnatsakanova A, Burchfiel CM. Police stressors and health: a state-of-the-art review. Policing: An International Journal of Police Strategies & Management. 2017;40(4):642-656. DOI: 10.1108/PIJPSM-06-2016-0097

[29] Nieuwenhuys A, Oudejans, RR. Anxiety and performance: perceptual-motor behavior in high-pressure contexts. Current Opinion in Psychology. Elsevier B.V. 2017;16:28-33. DOI:10.1016/j.copsyc.2017.03.019

[30] Covey TJ, Shucard JL, Violanti JM, Lee J, Shucard DW. The effects of exposure to traumatic stressors on inhibitory control in police officers: A dense electrode array study using a Go/NoGo continuous performance task. International Journal of Psychophysiology. 2013;87:363-375. DOI: 10.1016/j.ijpsycho.2013.03.009

[31] Clark JG, Jackson MS, Schaefer PM, Sharpe EG. Training SWAT teams: Implications for improving tactical units. Journal of Criminal Justice. 2000;28(5):407-413. DOI: 10.1016/S0047-2352(00)00055-6

[32] Williams JJ, Westall D. SWAT and non-SWAT police officers and the use of force. Journal of Criminal Justice. 2003;31(5):469-474. DOI: 10.1016/S0047-2352(03)00051-5

[33] Miller R, Stalder T, Jarczok M, Almeida DM, Badrick E, Bartels M, Boomsma DI, Coe CL, Dekker MC, Donzella B, Fischer JE. The CIRCORT database: reference ranges and seasonal changes in diurnal salivary cortisol derived from a meta-dataset comprised of 15 field studies. Psychoneuroendocrinology. 2016;73:16-23. DOI: 10.1016/j.psyneuen.2016.07.201

[34] McCreary DR, Fong I, Groll DL. Measuring police stress meaningfully: establishing norms and cut-off values for the operational and organizational police stress questionnaires. Police Pract Res. 2017; 18(6): 612-623. DOI:10.1080/15614263.2017.1363965

[35] CBC Docs POV. Police should be rewarded for community trust, not arrests, says expert [Internet]. 2020. Available from: https://www.cbc.ca/documentaries/cbc-docs-pov/police-should-be-rewarded-for-community-trust-not-arrests-says-expert-1.5635137 [Accessed: 2020-08-25]

[36] Burke D. Halifax police officers' crimes can erode public trust, says advocate. CBC [newspaper on the Internet]. 2019 Dec 2. Available from: https://www.cbc.ca/news/canada/nova-scotia/police-crime-accountability-mental-health-support-1.5374231 [Accessed: 2020-08-25]

[37] Thorn L, Hucklebridge F, Evans P, Clow A. The cortisol awakening response, seasonality, stress and arousal: a study of trait and state influences. Psychoneuroendocrinology. 2009 Apr 1;34(3):299-306. DOI: 10.1016/j.psyneuen.2008.11.005

[38] Andersen JP, Papazoglou K, Pitel M, Weerasinghe A, Daoust A. Predicting Police Performance from Stress Physiology: Implications for Police Training Policies. Poster Presentation at the 2016 Conference of the American Psychosomatic Society, Denver, CO.

[39] Joseph PN, Violanti JM, Donahue R, Andrew ME, Trevisan M, Burchfiel CM, Dorn J. Police work and subclinical atherosclerosis. Journal of Occupational and Environmental Medicine. 2009;51(6):700-707. DOI: 10.1097/JOM.0b013e3181a02252

[40] Violanti JM, Burchfiel CM, Miller DB, Andrew ME, Dorn J, Wactawski-Wende J, Beighley CM, Pierino K, Joseph PN, Vena JE, Sharp DS. The buffalo cardio-metabolic occupational police stress (BCOPS) pilot study: methods and participant characteristics. Annals of epidemiology. 2006;16(2):148-156. DOI: 10.1016/j.annepidem.2005.07.054

[41] Drogos LL, Wynne-Edwards K, Zhou R, Hall SE, Tyndall AV, Longman RS, Eskes G, Poulin MJ. Aerobic exercise increases cortisol awakening response in older adults. Psychoneuroendocrinology. 2019;103:241-248. DOI: 10.1016/j.psyneuen.2019.01.012

[42] Balthazar CH, Garcia MC, Spadari-Bratfisch RC. Salivary

concentrations of cortisol and testosterone and prediction of performance in a professional triathlon competition. Stress. 2012;15:495-502. DOI: 10.3109/10253890.2011.642033

[43] DeClerq K. Ontario police college no longer testing new recruits in physical fitness: memo. CTV News [newspaper on the Internet]. 2018 Sept 18. Available from: https://toronto.ctvnews.ca/ontario-police-college-no-longer-testing-new-recruits-in-physical-fitness-memo-1.4099292 [Accessed: 2020-08-25]

[44] Police Fitness Personnel Ontario. Ontario police fitness PIN award program [Internet]. 2013. Available from: http://www.pfpo.org/index.php/2013-01-12-19-00-53/ontario-police-fitness-pin-award-program [Accessed: 2020-08-25]

[45] CAMH. Police mental health: A discussion paper [Internet]. 2018. Available from: https://www.camh.ca/-/media/files/pdfs---public-policy-submissions/police-mental-health-discussion-paper-oct2018-pdf.pdf [Accessed: 2020-08-25]

Chapter 9

Modeling the Factors That Affect Work Accidents with Binary Logistic Regression: Evidence from Turkey

Ömer Alkan and Sena Gültekin

Abstract

Work accidents remain important worldwide. Work accidents and diseases influence the whole country economically, socially, and psychologically. The aim of this study was to determine the socio-demographic and economic factors that were influential for individuals in Turkey who experienced work accidents resulting in injuries. In this study, the Turkey Health Survey microdata set conducted by the Turkish Statistical Institute was employed including data from 35,019 employees who participated in the survey between 2008 and 2016. The factors affecting individuals' work accidents were determined by binary logistic regression analysis. According to analysis results, it was determined that the variables of gender, age, education, occupation, health, psycho-social support/being depressed, and use of alcohol have an impact on individuals having work accidents. Methods such as young employees receiving a good education, individuals completing their education before starting working, early intervention in diseases by regular employee check-ups, the reduction of stress in employees' working life, reduction of the negative effects of the job environment on employees, preservation of a healthy work-life balance, and supporting employees in their attempt to give up various bad habits such as smoking through rehabilitation can play significant roles in reducing work accidents.

Keywords: accident analysis, accident causes, employee, work accident, occupational safety, Turkey

1. Introduction

A work accident is defined as an accident that a worker suffers as a result of an incident that occurred suddenly due to an external reason for the work the worker performed for his employer while he was under the authority of the employer [1]. Before determining the causes of work accidents, the conditions that are accepted as being in the category of work accidents should be investigated. According to Law on Social Insurances and General Health Insurance No. 5510, the events that are accepted as work accidents are as follows: all accidents that include the period when the insured worker is in the workplace, the employee could not do his own job when he is sent to another place by the employer due to a job handled by the employer at the time, when female workers with small children are on maternity leave, and when the workers are collectively brought to another place by a vehicle provided by the employer [1].

Today, work accidents have become one of the most critical issues for our economy. The economic and psychological costs of these accidents have become a pressure factor in business life. Even if there is no accident, the constant risk to workers because of working conditions has become a major psychological problem [2].

The occurrence of accidents at workplaces and work-related diseases is of utmost importance in many respects such as protecting employee rights, fulfilling social responsibilities, and creating legal regulations. Although interest in work-related diseases began in the time of ancient Greece, work accidents and work-related diseases became an important issue during the Industrial Revolution and caused various labor movements and unionized employees to demand their rights. From the 19th century onwards, insurance companies began to offer insurance that covered work accidents and work-related diseases. In terms of Turkey, even though certain regulations had been in place since the 19th century in the Ottoman period, they were rather limited. After the establishment of the Republic of Turkey, laws were issued in limited areas, and then their scope was extended, covering all workers. To date, these laws have been updated many times, and improvements have been made [3].

Although technological developments have increased occupational health and safety, the alienation towards the job brought about by specialization, and a decreased sense of investment in the job has caused loss of attention during work which has led to work accidents. In this respect, creating a safe environment is of great importance in the working environment, but creating this environment is a rather difficult process because, apart from the current organization and working group, a safe climate appeals to individual perceptions [4]. In this context, it is also important to reduce stress in the working environment. There are studies indicating that work accidents increase as the level of stress increases in the work environment. In situations where stress, fear, and disgust are present, individuals experience more cognitive dysfunction and experience more accidents [5]. This damages the safety climate in the workplace. When a work accident occurs, workers cannot work efficiently because they are afraid for their own safety. For this reason, it is particularly important to provide an Occupational Health and Safety System in every workplace as well as to conduct studies on this issue [6].

Worldwide, 2.78 million workers die every year due to work accidents and work-related diseases. About 86.3% of these deaths are caused by work related diseases, and 13.7% are caused by work accidents. In non-fatal accidents, the number of injuries is higher. While for young workers it was determined that the accident rate was much higher, work-related diseases were lower. This situation stems from the situation of cumulative exposure to factors that cause work-related diseases and their delay time [7]. When work accidents were analyzed from a historical point of view, it was seen that they have regularly increased every year until 2010. There was a sharp decline in 2012, but later on an increase was observed. From 2012 to 2016 work accidents increased by 382%, and 84.29% of the people who experienced a work accident in 2016, were men [8].

When looking at the situation regarding work accidents in Turkey in 2016, it was seen that 32,52% of accidents and 60.85% of fatal accidents occurred in businesses that employed fewer than 50 people. More than half of the accidents occurred in working hours during the day, and 28.23% occurred before noon. The three industries that experienced the most work-related accidents in 2016 in Turkey were identified as factory-made metal product manufacturing except machinery and equipment, building construction, and specialized construction activities. These three industries made up 19.46% of all work accidents. In addition, the three industries where work accidents leading to fatalities occurred the most were building construction, land and pipeline transportation, and construction of outdoor buildings. The share of fatal work accidents in these three industries in the total volume of accidents was 39% [9].

The percentage of fatal accidents by economic activity per 100,000 workers in Turkey was divided into various business categories. Accordingly, while the highest accident rate occurred in agriculture, construction and sewage, waste management, and reclamation activities followed agriculture, respectively [8]. Worldwide, the construction industry has one of the highest occurrences of accidents. The use of large and heavy machinery and equipment increases the severity of injuries and the risk of death [10]. Although improvements have been made in developed countries, the construction sector in developing and under-developed countries is still one of the industries with the highest frequency of accidents [11].

According to the UCTEA (Union of Chambers of Turkish Engineers and Architects) report, in 2016, 20 people died on the first day of work, and 78 people died during the first week of work. While the number of people who died in the first eight to 30 days of the job, was up to 165 people, as experience increased, the number of people who had a fatal work accident decreased. 42.61% of workers involved in work accidents have 1 month to 1 year of experience at their job [9]. This situation shows how important experience and work proficiency are in work accidents [12]. When looking at the gender distribution in work accidents in general, it was determined that women had fewer accidents than men. However, in industries where women make up a higher percentage of employees, the manufacturing of food products, buildings and landscaping activities, and food and beverage service activities are the top three industries in which women experienced the most accidents in 2016 [13].

In a globalizing world, companies must improve their safety performance in order to compete on a global scale. Work accidents leading to permanent injuries, the accidents resulting in workers being unable to work for a long time, or the accident resulting in death create huge costs for companies. Investing in equipment to prevent work accidents and educating individuals in this area are important in terms of reducing costs. The development of a safety culture throughout the workplace is important in this context [14].

Many work accident and safety-related regulations have been made in Turkey in order to improve safety, and significant progress has been made. Labor Law No.1475 has been in force in Turkey since 1971, and it was amended in 2003 with Labor Law No. 4857. Since 2012, Occupational Health and Safety Law No. 6331 has been in force. Along with these laws, various improvements have been made in occupational health and safety. With the regulation issued in 2012, public and agricultural workers, as well as all workplaces and all employees regardless of the number of employees and the type of work, are covered within the scope of the law. In addition, risk assessment and increasing the number and capacity of occupational health and safety laboratories became compulsory for all businesses [8]. The National Occupational Health and Safety Council Regulation was issued in 2013. The aim of the council is to improve conditions related to safety in work life and to create a safety culture [15].

In spite of the arrangements made and the increase in precautions taken in Turkey in recent years, they are still far below the standards of developed countries. For this reason, many non-governmental organizations have been established, and these organizations have focused on issues such as increasing the legal rights of employees, improving working conditions, and workers being protected from harassment during the process after work accidents [16]. Although organizational safety is the responsibility of the employer, employees also have great responsibilities; they need to be careful and act consciously to prevent work accidents [14]. In this context, it is of great importance that employees use the protective gear prepared for them correctly, that they perform the emergency procedures that must be carried out in the event of an accident completely, and inform the proper authorities immediately–thus avoiding loss of lives [17].

Work accidents and diseases affect the whole country economically, socially and, psychologically. Work accidents constitute many cost elements such as lost working days, decrease in production, recruitment and training of new workers, compensation payments, and health expenditures. This situation causes state and company policies to be disrupted and sometimes not realized. In addition, the loss of human capital and the high budget share of social aid provided to the victims hinder new investments. From the perspective of the worker, the individual's loss of welfare, the psychological pressure, and loss of status that he and his family experience cause workers to feel as if they are a burden. In addition, accidents in the workplace also negatively affect other employees [6]. The aim of this study was to determine the socio-demographic and economic factors that are critical in individuals experiencing work accidents that result in injuries in Turkey. For this purpose, 10 factors were selected, and the impact of these factors on the probability of experiencing work accidents was examined. In this study, the Turkey Health Survey data made by the Turkish Statistical Institute (TSI) were employed.

2. Material and method

2.1 Data

The micro data set obtained from the Turkey Health Survey carried out by the TSI in 2008, 2010, 2012, 2014, and 2016 were used in this study. The Turkey Health Survey, which was first carried out in 2008, had been conducted every two years. The Turkey Health Survey was last conducted in 2016. With this survey, the aim is to minimize the information gap in the current structure by obtaining information for the health indicators that have a large share in the development indicators that show a country's level of development. In addition to being a survey that reflects the whole country, it is also important in enabling both international comparisons and shedding light on national needs. The scope of this survey is households that are located in all settlements within the borders of Turkey. Institutions including soldiers and permanent residents of dormitories, prison, nursing homes, hospitals, etc. are out of this survey's scope as well as locations (i.e. small villages, settlements of nomads, etc.) that are thought to be inadequate in terms of sample size (the number of population less than 20) have been excluded.

This survey was designed to give a total estimate for Turkey. A stratified two-stage cluster sampling method was used to obtain the data. The first stage sampling unit was randomly selected blocks from the clusters (blocks) containing an average of 100 household addresses with a proportionate stratification, and the second stage sampling unit was the household addresses systematically and randomly selected from each selected cluster [18–22].

In this study, the data from a total of 35,019 employees over 15 years old were employed, including 5473 people who participated in the Turkey Health Survey in 2008, 5238 people who participated in this survey in 2010, 10,436 people who participated in 2012, 7415 people who participated in 2014, and 6457 people who participated in 2016.

2.2 Measures and variables

The dependent variable of this study was a work accident of an individual measured by the question, "Have you had an accident that caused injury in the past 12 months?" The dependent variable was a binary variable. In the established binary logistic regression model, the dependent variable was categorized as 1 if the individual had had a work accident and 0 if not.

The independent variables are survey year (2008, 2010, 2012, 2014, 2016), gender (male, female), age group (15–24, 25–34, 35–44, 45–54, 55–64, 65+), education level (did not finish school/illiterate, primary school, secondary school, high school, university), marital status (single, married), work schedule (part-time, full time), profession (managers, professional occupational groups, technicians/assistant professional occupational groups, staff working in offices, service/sales staff, qualified agricultural/forestry/aquaculture workers, craftsmen/craft-related jobs, plant-machine operators/installers and those who work in jobs that do not require qualification), general health (very good/good, moderate, bad/very bad), psycho-social support/being depressed (no, yes), and alcohol use (no, yes). Ordinal and nominal variables were defined as dummy variables in order to observe the effects of the categories of all variables to be included in binary logistic regression model [23].

2.3 Research methodology

Survey statistics in Stata 15 (Stata Corporation) were used to account for the complex sampling design and weights. Weighted analysis was performed. First, frequency analyses of the variables in the model were performed. Then, chi-square independence tests were performed in order to detect the relationship between whether individuals had experienced a work accident and socio-economic and demographical factors. Last, factors which influenced the work accident experience of individuals were determined with binary logistic regression analysis.

3. Results

3.1 Descriptive statistics and chi-square test

Socio-demographic and economic factors that are critical in work-related accidents resulting in injury in Turkey are presented in **Table 1**.

19.2, 14.5, 28.9, 20, and 17.4% of those who experienced a work accident participated in the survey in 2008, 2010, 2012, 2014, and 2016, respectively. In terms of age range, 15.6% of employees who experienced work accidents were between 15 and 24 years old, 30.3% were between 25 and 34 years old, 29.2% were between 35 and 44 years old, 18.7% were between 45 and 54 years old, 4.5% were between 55 and 64 years old, and 1.8% were 65 years and older. In terms of education level, while 5.6% of workers, who had experienced work accidents were illiterate, 44.6% graduated from primary school, 21.4% were secondary school graduates, 20.3% were high school graduates, and 8.1% were university graduates. For occupational groups, while 3.2% of work accident victims were managers, 5.1% belonged to professional occupational groups, 5% were technicians and assistant members of professional occupations, 2.1% are office staff, 12.7% were service/sale staff, 15% were qualified agricultural/forestry/aquaculture workers, 26.9% were artists and related employees, 11.9% were facility-machinery operators/assemblers, and 18.1% were workers in non-qualified jobs.. While 67% of work accident victims had very good health, 26.3% had medium health, and 6.7%

Variables		Work Accident Experience		n (%)	P
		No	Yes		
Survey year	2008	5271 (15.5)	202 (19.2)	5473 (15.6)	0.033[b]
	2010	5085 (15.0)	153 (14.5)	5238 (15.0)	
	2012	10,131 (29.8)	305 (28.9)	10,436 (29.8)	
	2014	7204 (21.2)	211 (20.0)	7415 (21.2)	
	2016	6274 (18.5)	183 (17.4)	6457 (18.4)	
Gender	Female	9885 (29.1)	159 (15.1)	10,044 (28.7)	0.000[a]
	Male	24,080 (70.9)	895 (84.9)	24,975 (71.3)	
Age	15–24	3757 (11.1)	164 (15.6)	3921 (11.2)	0.000[a]
	25-34	9478 (27.9)	319 (30.3)	9797 (28.0)	
	35–44	9978 (29.4)	308 (29.2)	10,286 (29.4)	
	45–54	6913 (20.4)	197 (18.7)	7110 (20.3)	
	55–64	2790 (8.2)	47 (4.5)	2837 (8.1)	
	65+	1049 (3.1)	19 (1.8)	1068 (3.0)	
Level of education	Did not finish school/illiterate	2183 (6.4)	59 (5.6)	2242 (6.4)	0.000[a]
	Primary school	11,985 (35.3)	470 (44.6)	12,455 (35.6)	
	Secondary school	5104 (15.0)	226 (21.4)	5330 (15.2)	
	High school	7093 (20.9)	214 (20.3)	7307 (20.9)	
	University	7600 (22.4)	85 (8.1)	7685 (21.9)	
Marital status	Single	8040 (23.7)	266 (25.2)	8306 (23.7)	0.239
	Married	25,925 (76.3)	788 (74.8)	26,713 (76.3)	
Work schedule	Part-time	2078 (6.1)	55 (5.2)	2133 (6.1)	0.229
	Full time	31,887 (93.9)	999 (94.8)	32,886 (93.9)	
Occupation	Manager	2459 (7.2)	34 (3.2)	2493 (7.1)	0.000[a]
	Professional occupation group	4815 (14.2)	54 (5.1)	4869 (13.9)	
	Technician	2502 (7.4)	53 (5.0)	2555 (7.3)	
	Office worker	1980 (5.8)	22 (2.1)	2002 (5.7)	
	Service employee and sale representative	5456 (16.1)	134 (12.7)	5590 (16.0)	
	Qualified agricultural worker	5164 (15.2)	158 (15.0)	5322 (15.2)	
	Artist	4659 (13.7)	283 (26.9)	4942 (14.1)	
	Equipment and machinery operator	2807 (8.3)	125 (11.9)	2932 (8.4)	
	Non-qualified job worker	4123 (12.1)	191 (18.1)	4314 (12.3)	
General Health	Very Good	25,153 (74.1)	706 (67.0)	25,859 (73.9)	0.000[a]
	Medium	7276 (21.4)	277 (26.3)	7553 (21.6)	
	Very Poor	1529 (4.5)	71 (6.7)	1600 (4.6)	

Variables		Work Accident Experience		n (%)	P
		No	Yes		
Psycho-social support/ depression	No	32,078 (94.4)	969 (91.9)	33,047 (94.4)	0.001[a]
	Yes	1887 (5.6)	85 (8.1)	1972 (5.6)	
Alcohol use	No	25,862 (76.1)	766 (72.7)	26,628 (76.0)	0.009[a]
	Yes	8103 (23.9)	288 (27.3)	8391 (24.0)	

[a] $p < .01$
[b] $p < .05$.

Table 1.
Distribution of factors that affect whether individuals experience work accidents.

had extremely poor health. In addition, 8.1% of work accident victims had received psycho-social support or were depressed. Finally, 27.3% of work accident victims drank alcohol.

According to the chi-square independence test results in **Table 1**, a significant relationship was found between individuals experiencing work accidents with injury and socio-demographic and economic variables (except marital status and work schedule).

3.2 Model estimation

Variance Inflation Factors (VIF) value, β coefficient, standard error, OR value, and confidence intervals related to the binary logistic regression model are shown in **Table 2**. Before model estimation, the issue of multicollinearity between variables should be investigated. Variables with a VIF value over five caused mid-level multicollinearity, and variables with a VIF value over 10 caused high multicollinearity [24]. As seen in **Table 2**, no variable in the model has a VIF value of five or above. Accordingly, no variable that causes multicollinearity between variables in the model exists.

According to the binary logistic regression analysis, when OR < 1, the estimated factor (according to the reference category) had little effect on the investigated state. When OR > 1, it had an increasing effect compared to the reference category [25]. As a result of the analysis, compared to the individuals surveyed in 2008, the odds ratio of individuals who participated in the survey in 2014 (OR = 0.770; 95% CI = 0.615–0.964) and 2016 (OR = 0.782; 95% CI = 0.617–0.991), was lower. In addition, men (OR = 2.246; 95% CI = 1.822–2.769) had higher odds of having a work accident than women. Considering the age variable, compared to the 15–24 group, the age ranges of 25–34 (OR = 0.795; 95% CI = 0.611–1.035), 35–44 (OR = 0.601; 95% CI = 0.450–0.803), 45–54 (OR = 0.486; 95% CI = 0.355–0.665), 55–64 (OR = 0.300; 95% CI = 0.197–0.458) and 65+ (OR = 0.296; 95% CI = 0.162–0.542) had a lower odds ratio of experiencing work accidents.

In terms of educational status, it was seen that primary school graduates (OR = 1.714; 95% CI = 1.208–2.434), secondary school graduates (OR = 1.554; 95% CI = 1.087–2.222), and high school graduates (OR = 1.612; 95% CI = 1.160–2.238) had higher odds ratio of work accident than university graduates. When the occupational groups were examined, technicians/assistant professional members (OR = 2.008; 95% CI = 1.225–3.292), service/sales staff (OR = 1.848; 95% CI = 1.189–2.875), qualified agriculture/forestry/aquaculture workers (OR = 3.031; 95% CI = 1.922–4.781), craftsmen/related workers (OR = 4.270;

Variables	VIF	β	Std. Error	P	OR	95% CI	
						Low.	Up.
Survey year (reference category: 2008)							
2010	1.67	-0.195	0.122	0.111	0.823	0.648	1.046
2012	2.09	-0.128	0.104	0.219	0.880	0.717	1.079
2014	1.9	-0.261	0.114	0,022[b]	0.770	0.615	0.964
2016	1.85	-0.246	0.121	0,042[b]	0.782	0.617	0.991
Gender (reference category: female)							
Male	1.2	0.809	0.107	0.000[a]	2.246	1.822	2.769
Age (reference category: 15–24)							
25–34	3.25	-0.229	0.134	0.088[c]	0.795	0.611	1.035
35–44	3.90	-0.509	0.148	0.001[a]	0.601	0.450	0.803
45–54	3.39	-0.721	0.160	0.000[a]	0.486	0.355	0.665
55–64	2.19	-1.202	0.215	0.000[a]	0.300	0.197	0.458
65+	1.56	-1.217	0.308	0.000[a]	0.296	0.162	0.542
Level of education (reference category: university)							
Did not finish school/illiterate	1.89	0.339	0.230	0.141	1.404	0.894	2.204
Primary school	3.25	0.539	0.179	0.003[a]	1.714	1.208	2.434
Secondary school	2.16	0.441	0.182	0.016[b]	1.554	1.087	2.222
High school	2.00	0.477	0.168	0.004[a]	1.612	1.160	2.238
Marital status (reference category: single)							
Married	1.53	0.079	0.109	0.467	1.082	0.875	1.339
Work schedule (reference category: part time)							
Full time	1.06	0.072	0.168	0.669	1.074	0.773	1.494
Occupation (reference category: manager)							
Professional occupational group worker	2.87	0.440	0.267	0.100	1.553	0.920	2.624
Technician	1.91	0.697	0.252	0.006[a]	2.008	1.225	3.292
Office worker	1.76	-0.007	0.313	0.982	0.993	0.538	1.833
Service employee and sale representative	2.87	0.614	0.225	0.006[a]	1.848	1.189	2.875
Qualified agricultural worker	3.15	1.109	0.233	0.000[a]	3.031	1.922	4.781
Artist	2.78	1.452	0.218	0.000[a]	4.270	2.786	6.542
Facility and machinery operator	2.11	1.020	0.228	0.000[a]	2.774	1.773	4.340
Non-qualified job worker	2.65	1.241	0.224	0.000[a]	3.459	2.228	5.370
General health status (reference category: poor)							
Very good	4.97	-0.650	0.154	0.000[a]	0.522	0.386	0.706

Variables	VIF	β	Std. Error	P	OR	95% CI	
						Low.	Up.
Medium	4.61	−0.242	0.155	0.120	0.785	0.579	1.065
Psycho-social support/depression (reference category: no)							
Yes	1.05	0.495	0.140	0.000[a]	1.641	1.246	2.160
Alcohol use (reference category: no)							
Yes	1.09	0.286	0.084	0.001[a]	1.331	1.130	1.568

VIF, variance inflation factor; Std. Error, standard error; Low., lower; Up., upper.
[a]*p < .01*
[b]*p < .05*
[c]*p < .10.*

Table 2.
Binary logistic regression estimation results of socio-demographic and economic factors that affect whether individuals experience work accidents.

95% CI = 2.786–6.542), plant-machine operators/assemblers (OR = 2.774; 95% CI = 1.773–4.340), and those who work in jobs that do not require qualification (OR = 3.459; 95% CI = 2.228–5.370) have higher odds of having a work accident than managers. When general health status is examined, the odds ratio of experiencing work accident of those with very good health (OR = 0.522; 95% CI = 0.386–0.706) is lower than those with poor health status. People who receive psycho-social support/ are depressed (OR = 1.641; 95% CI = 1.246–2.160) had higher odds of having a work accident than others. Finally, the odds ratio of experiencing work accidents for participants who used alcohol (OR = 1.331; 95% CI = 1.130–1.568) was higher than for those who did not.

3.3 Average direct elasticity

Average direct elasticities and standard errors in the socio-demographic and economic factors that influence whether individuals experience work accidents resulting in injuries in Turkey are provided in **Table 3**.

For marginal effects, the probability of experiencing work accidents was lower in other years compared to 2008. In terms of gender, the probability of men experiencing work accidents was 78.9% higher than women. Also, as age increased compared to the age range of 15–24, the probability of work accidents decreased. The probability of individuals within the age groups of 25–34, 35–44, 45–54, 55–64, and 65+ are 22%, 49%, 69,6%, 116,8% and 118,2%, respectively, lower than the 15–24 age range.

When the education levels are analyzed, primary school graduates, secondary school graduates, and high school graduates are 52.4%, 42.9%, and 46.5% more likely to have a work accident than university graduates, respectively.

When looking at the occupational groups, the probability of technicians, service/sales staff, qualified agricultural workers, craftsmen, plant/machine operators, and those who do not work in qualified jobs is, respectively, 68.5, 60.4, 108.4, 141, 99.9, and 121.1% higher than managers.

When the general health status is examined, those with very good general health status are 62.4% less likely to have a work accident than those who have poor health. In addition, those who receive psycho-social support/are depressed are 47.6% more likely to have a work accident than other individuals. Those who use alcohol are 27.6% more likely to have a work accident than those who do not.

Variables	Elasticity (%)	Std. Error
Year (reference category: 2008)		
2010	−18.8	0.118
2012	**−12.4**	**0.100**
2014	−25.3[b]	0.111
2016	−23.8[b]	0.117
Gender (reference category: female)		
Male	78.9[a]	0.105
Age (reference category: 15–24)		
25–34	−22.0[c]	0.128
35–44	−49.0[a]	0.142
45-54	−69.6[a]	0.154
55-64	−116.8[a]	0.21
65+	−118.2[a]	0.302
Level of education (reference category: university)		
Did not finish school/illiterate	33.1	0.224
Primary school	52.4[a]	0.175
Secondary school	42.9[b]	0.178
High school	46.5[a]	0.164
Marital status (reference category: single)		
Married	7.7	0.105
Work schedule (reference category: part time)		
Full time	7.0	0.163
Occupation (reference category: manager)		
Professional occupational group worker	43.4	0.263
Technician	68.5[a]	0.248
Office worker	−0.71	0.309
Service employee and sale representative	60.4[a]	0.222
Qualified agricultural worker	108.4[a]	0.228
Artist	141.2[a]	0.214
Facility and machinery operator	99.9[a]	0.244
Non-qualified Job worker	121.1[a]	0.221
General health status (reference category: poor)		
Very good	−62.4[a]	0.146
Medium	−23.1	0.148
Psycho-social support/depression (reference category: no)		
Yes	47,6[a]	0.134
Alcohol use (reference category: no)		
Yes	27,6[a]	0.081

Std. Error, standard error.
[a]$p < .01$.
[b]$p < .05$.
[c]$p < .10$.

Table 3.
Elasticity estimates for socio-demographic and economic factors that influence whether individuals experience work accidents.

4. Discussion

Work accidents remain important worldwide. Work accidents and diseases influence the whole country economically, socially, and psychologically. 286.068 work accidents occurred in Turkey in 2016. 1405 people died in these work accidents [9]. The loss of these people exerted great pressure on the country, both socially and economically. In addition, even if these accidents did not result in loss of life, the workers being unable to work as a result of their injuries, their inability to continue their work for a long time, or scars they have because of these accidents psychologically depress individuals, apart from economic problems. For this reason, it is of great importance to determine the causes of work accidents and to try to prevent these accidents by concentrating on their causes [6].

The aim of this study was to investigate the factors affecting work accidents of individuals that resulted in injuries in the last 12 months in which the survey was conducted in Turkey. As a result of the analysis, the variables of gender, age, education, occupation, health, psycho-social support/depression, and alcohol use were detected statistically significant.

According to study findings, men have more work accidents than women. Similar results can be found in many studies in the literature [26, 27]. In addition, it was detected in some studies that men are more likely to experience fatal work accidents [28]. This situation can be explained with the fact that men work more in dangerous jobs that require physical power than women.

According to the results of the analysis, it was found that the age range that had the most work accidents was 25–34, while the age range that had the least accidents was 65+. Although the physical activity of workers decreased as they get older, their increased experience was effective in decreasing work accidents with age. In this context, there are many studies showing that work accidents are most common in the 25–44 age range and least common in the 65+ age range [12, 13, 29–31]. In some studies, the 16–24 age range was found to be the age group where work accidents occurred most frequently [26, 32]. There are also studies indicating that the 35–45 age range is the age group that most frequently experiences fatal work accidents [28].

It was detected that the probability of having a work accident decreases with an increase in the level of education. This may be due to the fact that workers who have a low level of education work in low-profile and risky jobs, or it may be due to individuals having an incomplete understanding risk factors due to a lack of education [31, 33, 34]. In addition, individuals who had not received vocational training were more likely to experience work accidents. Therefore, individuals should undergo specific training before starting to work, and, basic work-related safety measures should be taught [35]. In addition, the fact that individuals did not have sufficient work-related training increased the risk of fatal accidents. One out of every five deaths in construction workers and 95% of the deceased workers were uneducated people [28]. Workers receiving professional training to improve their job competencies and increase their job-related knowledge had an important role in preventing work accidents. In addition, developing a safety culture with training activities and the integration of these activities into corporate culture will make safety a reality at each level [36]. Also, as job safety and health training become more appealing, individuals will receive three times more information, thus considerably reducing work accidents. Applied, student-centered, and participatory training activities should be therefore put into practice [37].

It was detected that individuals working in lower level jobs were more exposed to work accidents. This may arise from the risk and safety awareness of the employees. It is expected that this result arises from the fact that those who work in jobs requiring more strength have generally received less education and people who work in upper-level positions, such as managers, will have a certain awareness, due to their education. There is a strong relationship between safety awareness and risks experienced [38]. For this reason, improving the safety awareness of individuals is of utmost importance. Accordingly, it is vital that individuals receive training in risk management and the use of personal protective equipment [39].

It was detected in the study that people who had received psycho-social support/had experienced depression had more work accidents. It has been demonstrated in several studies that stressful living conditions increase the probability of having a work accident. It has been demonstrated that situations affecting the personal life of individuals, such as being unable to consume adequate food, a suffocating work life, and environmental problems, increase the risk of work accidents [33, 40–42]. Stress and pressure can have different consequences on the probability of men or women to experience work accidents. While stress caused by a lack of organizational support in women is a major reason for them to experience work accidents, this situation was not applicable to men experiencing work accidents [43]. Accordingly, individuals' low level of social support from their workplace and stress increased work accidents. It has also been reported in similar studies that women are more affected by workload and stress [44, 45]. However, the fact that individuals experience the pressure of the requirements of high productivity also increases the likelihood of work accidents because individuals can display dangerous behaviors due to this pressure [46]. All these behaviors and stress trigger further depression.

5. Conclusions

According to the study results, alcohol consumption caused an increased rate of work accidents. There are studies that demonstrate alcohol use and smoking increase work accidents, both in men and women [44]. Contrary to this study, there are also other studies in the literature demonstrating that bad habits such as using alcohol and smoking do not influence work accidents [45]. Additionally, it was found that people with poor health are more likely to experience work accidents than people with good health. In general, people's poor health conditions make them unable to focus on their job and not being careful enough. This situation leads employees to being exposed to accidents.

Methods such as young employees receiving a good education, workers completing their education before beginning work, regular check-ups for employees and early intervention in diseases, attempts to reduce stress in work life as well as to reduce the negative impact of the job environment on employees, preserving a positive work-life balance, and supporting employees with bad habits such as alcohol and smoking through various rehab activities can play significant roles in reducing work accidents. Also, having first aid experts and doctors constantly available on the job site will help to minimize bad outcome from injuries with early intervention in accidents. In addition, workers not working for long hours during the day, workers having sufficient breaks, and workers having holidays will prevent loss of focus during work, thus playing a great role in reducing work accidents. Using safety signs in workplaces, having constant supervision of employees during working hours, and immediate intervention with people who violate safety rules will have a minimizing impact on work accidents.

6. Limitations

This study had several limitations. First, the study data were secondary data. Variables required for statistical analysis consisted of existing variables in the dataset. Second, as the data was cross-sectional, a definitive causal relationship on factors that influence work accidents could not be inferred. Third, this study was not based on recorded data. The data were collected through surveys conducted by the TSI. The data obtained in this study were direct responses from individuals. Since there is no officially recorded data, results obtained from the data collection method could be biased. Fourth, since the data was collected via a survey and actively answered by working individuals, it did not contain data related to fatal accidents. Finally, the frequency of alcohol consumption for individuals who drank alcohol could not be determined.

Acknowledgements

The authors would like to thank the Turkish Statistical Institute for the data. The views and opinions expressed in this manuscript are those of the authors only and do not necessarily represent the views, official policy, or position of the Turkish Statistical Institute.

Funding

This research did not receive any specific grant from funding agencies in the public, commercial, or not-for-profit sectors.

Conflict of interest

The authors declare no conflict of interest.

Author details

Ömer Alkan* and Sena Gültekin
Ataturk University, Erzurum, Turkey

*Address all correspondence to: oalkan@atauni.edu.tr

References

[1] HAK-İŞ, ÇASGEM. Sosyal Diyalog Yoluyla Kadın Dostu İş Yerlerini Belgelendirme Projesi: Kadın Çalışanlar İçin İSG Rehberi, 2016, Başak Matbaası: Hak-İş Konfederasyonu, Ankara

[2] ILO. Çalışma yaşamının geleceğinin merkezinde sağlık ve güvenlik: 100 yıllık deneyimden hareketle, 2019, Uluslararası Çalışma Örgütü Ankara.

[3] Çetindağ Ş. İş sağlığı ve güvenliği'nin tarihsel gelişimi ve mevzuattaki güncel durum. Toprak İşveren Dergisi. 2010; 86:26-28.

[4] Leitão S, Greiner BA. Organisational safety climate and occupational accidents and injuries: an epidemiology-based systematic review. Work & Stress. 2016; 30(1):71-90.

[5] Wallace JC, Chen G. Development and validation of a work-specific measure of cognitive failure: Implications for occupational safety. Journal of Occupational and Organizational Psychology. 2005; 78(4):615-632.

[6] Kılkış İ. İş sağlığı ve güvenliği, in Sosyal politika, A. Tokol and Y. Alper, Editors. Dora yayınları: Bursa;2011; 194-220.

[7] ILO. Genç işçilerin sağlık ve güvenliğinin iyileştirilmesi, 2018, Uluslararası Çalışma Örgütü Ankara.

[8] Bilir N. İş sağlığı ve güvenliği profili Türkiye, 2016, Uluslararası Çalışma Örgütü (ILO): Ankara.

[9] TMMOB. İş Sağlığı ve Güvenliği Oda Raporu, Yayın No: MMO/689, 2018, Türkiye Makine Mühendisleri Odası Ankara.

[10] Abudayyeh O, Fredericks TK, Butt SE, Shaar A. An investigation of management's commitment to construction safety. International Journal of Project Management. 2006; 24(2):167-174.

[11] Awwad R, El Souki O, Jabbour M. Construction safety practices and challenges in a Middle Eastern developing country. Safety Science. 2016; 83:1-11.

[12] Ghasemi F, Kalatpour O, Moghimbeigi A, Mohammadfam I. Selecting strategies to reduce high-risk unsafe work behaviors using the safety behavior sampling technique and Bayesian network analysis. Journal of Research in Health Sciences. 2017; 17(1):1-6.

[13] Altunkaynak B. A statistical study of occupational accidents in the manufacturing industry in Turkey. International Journal of Industrial Ergonomics. 2018; 66:101-109.

[14] Beriha G, Patnaik B, Mahapatra S, Padhee S. Assessment of safety performance in Indian industries using fuzzy approach. Expert Systems with Applications. 2012; 39(3):3311-3323.

[15] Resmigazete. Ulusal İş Sağlığı Ve Güvenliği Konseyi Yönetmeliği, Ç.v.S.G. Bakanlığı, Editor 2013: Ankara.

[16] Akin L. Sendikaların iş sağlığı ve güvenliğinin sağlanmasına katkısı. Calisma ve Toplum. 2012; 34(3):101-123.

[17] Demirbilek T, Çakır Ö. Kişisel koruyucu donanim kullanimini etkileyen bireysel ve örgütsel değişkenler. Dokuz Eylül Üniversitesi İktisadi İdari Bilimler Fakültesi Dergisi. 2008; 23(2):173-191.

[18] TUİK. Turkey Health Survey Micro Data Set, 2008. 2008 15.04.2020]; Available from: http://www.tuik.gov.tr/

MicroVeri/sagAr_2008/english/index.html.

[19] TUİK. Turkey Health Survey Micro Data Set, 2010. 2010 15.04.2020]; Available from: http://www.tuik.gov.tr/MicroVeri/sagAr_2010/english/index.html.

[20] TUİK. Turkey Health Survey Micro Data Set, 2012. 2012 15.04.2020]; Available from: http://www.tuik.gov.tr/MicroVeri/sagAr_2012/english/index.html.

[21] TUİK. Turkey Health Survey Micro Data Set, 2014. 2014 15.04.2020]; Available from: http://www.tuik.gov.tr/MicroVeri/sagAr_2014/english/index.html.

[22] TUİK. Turkey Health Survey Micro Data Set, 2016. 2016 15.04.2020]; Available from: http://www.tuik.gov.tr/MicroVeri/sagAr_2016/english/index.html.

[23] Alkan Ö, Abar H. Determination of factors influencing tobacco consumption in Turkey using categorical data analyses1. Archives of Environmental & Occupational Health. 2020; 75(1):27-35.

[24] Alkan Ö. Türkiye'de gençlerin tütün kullanımında cinsiyet farklılıklarının araştırılması. Bağımlılık Dergisi. 2017; 18(2):35-45.

[25] Alkan Ö, Demir A. Tütün kullanımını bırakma başarısını etkileyen faktörlerin lojistik regresyon ile analizi. Ataturk University Journal of Economics & Administrative Sciences. 2019; 33(4):1227-1244.

[26] Nghitanwa EM, Lindiwe Z. Occupational accidents and injuries among workers in the construction industry of Windhoek, Namibia. International Journal of Health. 2017; 5(1):55-59.

[27] Hansen CD. Comparing fatal occupational accidents in Denmark and Sweden 1993-2012. Occupational Medicine. 2019; 69(4):283-286.

[28] Ling FYY, Liu M, Woo YC. Construction fatalities in Singapore. International Journal of Project Management. 2009; 27(7):717-726.

[29] Macedo AC, Silva IL. Analysis of occupational accidents in Portugal between 1992 and 2001. Safety Science. 2005; 43(5-6):269-286.

[30] Unsar S, Sut N. General assessment of the occupational accidents that occurred in Turkey between the years 2000 and 2005. Safety Science. 2009; 47(5):614-619.

[31] Alizadeh SS, Mortazavi SB, Sepehri MM. Analysis of occupational accident fatalities and injuries among male group in Iran between 2008 and 2012. Iranian Red Crescent Medical Journal. 2015; 17(10):e18976.

[32] Berglund L, Johansson M, Nygren M, Samuelson B, Stenberg M, Johansson J. Occupational accidents in Swedish construction trades. International Journal of Occupational Safety and Ergonomics. 2019:1-10.

[33] Barlas B, Izci FB. Individual and workplace factors related to fatal occupational accidents among shipyard workers in Turkey. Safety Science. 2018; 101:173-179.

[34] Aliabadi MM, Aghaei H. Analysis of the severity of occupational injuries in the mining industry using a Bayesian network. Epidemiology and Health. 2019; 41:e2019017.

[35] Lette A, Ambelu A, Getahun T, Mekonen S. A survey of work-related injuries among building construction workers in southwestern Ethiopia. International Journal of Industrial Ergonomics. 2018; 68:57-64.

[36] Ren J, Jenkinson I, Wang J, Xu D, Yang J. A methodology to model causal relationships on offshore safety assessment focusing on human and organizational factors. Journal of Safety Research. 2008; 39(1):87-100.

[37] Burke MJ, Sarpy SA, Smith-Crowe K, Chan-Serafin S, Salvador RO, Islam G. Relative effectiveness of worker safety and health training methods. American Journal of Public Health. 2006; 96(2):315-324.

[38] Akalp G, Aytac S, Yamankaradeniz N, Cankaya O, Gokce A, Tufekci U. Perceived safety culture and occupational risk factors among women in metal industries: A study in Turkey. Procedia Manufacturing. 2015; 3:4956-4963.

[39] Zhang G, Thai VV, Law AWK, Yuen KF, Loh HS, Zhou Q. Quantitative risk assessment of seafarers' nonfatal injuries due to occupational accidents based on bayesian network modeling. Risk Analysis. 2020; 40(1):8-23.

[40] Cordeiro R, Dias A. Stressful life events and occupational accidents. Scandinavian Journal of Work, Environment & Health. 2005; 31(5):336-342.

[41] Day AJ, Brasher K, Bridger RS. Accident proneness revisited: the role of psychological stress and cognitive failure. Accident Analysis & Prevention. 2012; 49:532-535.

[42] Barkhordari A, Malmir B, Malakoutikhah M. An analysis of individual and social factors affecting occupational accidents. Safety and Health at Work. 2019; 10(2):205-212.

[43] Julià M, Catalina-Romero C, Calvo-Bonacho E, Benavides FG. The impact of job stress due to the lack of organisational support on occupational injury. Occupational and Environmental Medicine. 2013; 70(9):623-629.

[44] Wilkins K, Mackenzie SG. Work injuries. Health Rep. 2007; 18(3):25-42.

[45] Kim HC, Min JY, Min KB, Park SG. Job strain and the risk for occupational injury in small-to medium-sized manufacturing enterprises: A prospective study of 1,209 Korean employees. American Journal of Industrial Medicine. 2009; 52(4):322-330.

[46] Mearns K, Flin R, Gordon R, Fleming M. Human and organizational factors in offshore safety. Work & Stress. 2001; 15(2):144-160.

Chapter 10

Occupational Heat Stress: A Technical Scan

Krishnan Srinivasan, Smisha Mohan and Jeneth Berlin Raj T

Abstract

The trouble for every person is to competently interact with his/her environmental variables. India being a tropical country will have a huge impact on individuals' health as a result of this global warming. Workers who are working in a hot environment pose an extra risk as they are exposed to additional heat in the workplace. The diversity in Indian climatic systems necessitates scientific study in different regions of the country. Methods to quantify the heat strain vary in different countries & different professional groups. Most of the previous studies on assessing the health effects have been conducted on simulation settings rather than actual field settings. Research in occupational heat stress is much needed to find out the health impacts and suitable intervention to protect workers health which subsequently reduces the morbidity.

Keywords: climate change, occupational heat stress, heat strain, prevention, adaptive measures

1. Introduction

The current prediction on climate change says that there will be an increase in the ambient temperature of about 0.5 to 1 degree C by 2030 which may pose a significant risk to the people [1, 2]. India being a tropical country will have a huge impact on individuals' health as a result of this global warming [2]. Workers who are working in a hot environment pose an extra risk as they are exposed to additional heat in the workplace [3]. Occupational heat stress is the net heat load experienced by the worker which includes the combined contributions of metabolic heat produced during the time of work, environmental factors, and clothing [4]. Continuous exposure to excessive heat may result in heat-related illness which ranges from heat rash to heat stroke which life is threatening. Apart from this the workers are at increased risk of accidents at workplaces, decreased productivity which all can cause an increase in morbidity and decrease in community economy. Various factors play a major role in determining the heat stress which includes ambient temperature, humidity, air movement, source of heat, duration of exposure, fluid loss/intake, etc. [5]. Indoor and outdoor workers are at risk of heat stress. Occupational heat stress will cause potential negative health with wellbeing outcome. In this chapter, the basics of occupational heat stress and heat strain, physiology thermoregulation, vulnerable population group, health impacts, Current status of research in occupational heat stress, prevention, control and adaptive measures will be discussed. To achieve this, a technical scan of various research papers pertaining to heat stress that were published in the last ten years were considered and the key points are included in this chapter.

2. What is occupational heat stress?

Heat stress includes many physical reactions that result from a body's capacity to regulate its temperature in response to the environment [6, 7]. Failure in the body regulatory mechanism will lead to heat stress which may cause increase in core body temperature and heat rate. This may further cause accumulation of excess heat in the body which cause the worker to lose concentration in working environment and may become irritable or sick [8]. High air temperatures, radiant heat sources, high humidity, direct physical contact with hot objects, and strenuous physical activities may cause increase risk of developing heat related illness.

Occupational heat stress is that the net load to which a worker is exposed from the combined contributions of metabolic heat, environmental factors, and clothing worn which leads to rise in heat storage within the body [1]. Workers who are working in hot environment are at increased risk of developing heat related illness. Heat stress results in heat related illness and also it may account for an increase in workplace accidents, and a decrease in worker productivity [7, 9]. Heat stress related health impacts ranges from less severe heat rash to more severe heat stroke. Sweaty palms, fogged-up safety glasses and dizziness are the main causes for workplace injury. Burns may also occur as a result of accidental contact with hot surfaces or steam [6, 10]. In India occupational heat stress is becoming more significant as the average temperatures increase but remains overlooked [3, 11, 12]. Both indoor and outdoor workers are at risk of developing heat related illness. Outdoor work sector includes agriculture, construction, brick industry where as indoor work includes firefighters, bakery workers, farmers, miners, boiler room workers, factory workers [12, 13].

3. Physiology of thermoregulation

The internal temperature (Core) of healthy human body should be maintained around 37°C for the various metabolic processes to function at optimum range inside the human body [14]. Variations, usually of less than 1°C occur with the time of the day, level of physical activity or emotional state [15]. As the environment warms-up, the body tends to warm-up as well. In this way, the body increases the rate of heat loss to balance the heat burden created by the environment. In a very hot environment, the rate of heat gain exceeds the rate of heat loss and the body temperature begins to rise. There are number of physiological heat control mechanisms playing a vital role in maintaining the core body temperature even when the external air temperature is greater than 37° C [16]. The pre-optic area in the anterior hypothalamus of the brain along with posterior hypothalamus, medulla, pons and spinal cord maintain core body temperature within normal range. The thermal sensors maintain a constant core body temperature by increasing blood flow to the skin (Vasodilatation) and by increasing sweat production [15]. To balance the heat burden created by the environment, the body increases the rate of heat loss. A rise in the body temperature results in heat related illnesses [17].

The main source of heat gain in a human body is production of its own internal heat called metabolic heat. It is generated within the body by the biochemical processes that keep us alive and by the energy we use during physical activity. The body exchanges heat with its surroundings mainly through radiation, convection, and evaporation of sweat [6]. Radiation is the process by which the body gains heat from surrounding hot objects, such as hot metal, furnaces or steam pipes and lose heat to objects such as chilled metallic surfaces without contact with them [14]. Convection is the process by which the body exchanges heat with the surrounding air. The body gains heat from hot air and loses heat to cold air which comes in contact with the skin. Convective heat exchange increases with increasing air speed and increased differences between air and skin temperature [14]. The body cools as the evaporation of sweat from the skin occurs. Evaporation sets in very quickly and effect is more enhanced with high wind speeds and low relative humidity. In hot and dry workplaces, the cooling due to sweat evaporation is limited by the amount of sweat produced by the body [6].

The body also exchanges small amounts of heat by conduction and breathing. By conduction the body gain or lose heat when it comes into direct contact with hot or cold objects. Breathing exchanges heat because the respiratory system warms the inhaled air. The body's excess heat is pushed away as the exhalation sets in. However, the amount of heat exchanged through conduction and breathing is normally small enough to be ignored in assessing the heat load on the body [18].

4. Heat stress and heat strain indicators

There are many indices that are used to assess heat stress such asWet bulb Globe Thermometer (WBGT), Universal Thermal Climate Index, Humidex, etc. WBGT is the gold standard internationally accepted indices for measuring heat stress and it was used to measure the heat stress in most of the previous research work conducted in different occupational sectors [19] (**Figure 1**).

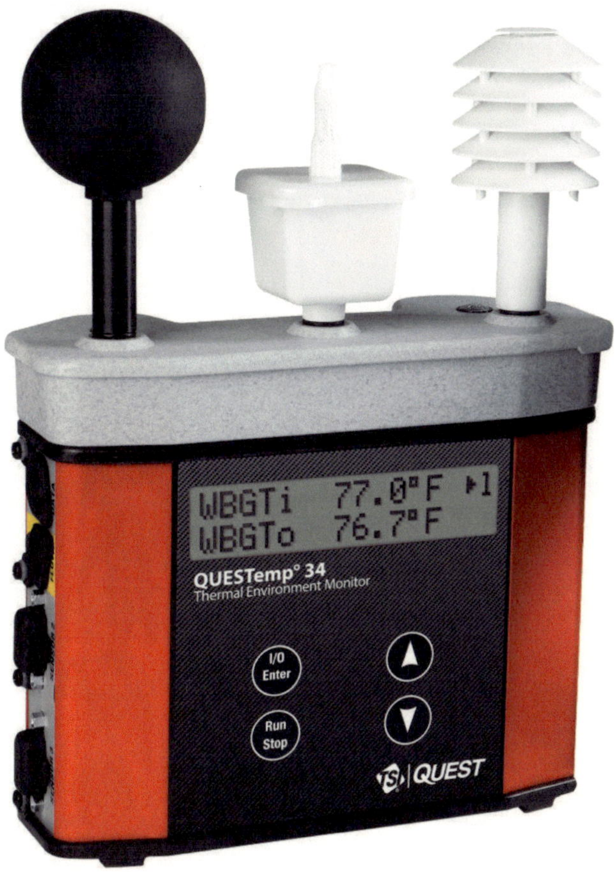

Figure 1.
WBGT.

A wide range of clinical observations and measurement have been used to indicate heat strain, ranging from perception of workers, observational parameter like skin rash to hospitalization due to heat stroke. Most of the previous studies on assessing the health effects have been conducted on simulation settings rather than actual field settings. Such studies although provides us with important information on the relationship, it might not be possible to use the same methodology at work place. The heat strain parameters that were measured in the previous studies include core body temperature [20], Skin temperature [14], Sweat rate [21], Resting/working heart rate [22], Urinary specific gravity [23], Serum creatinine, Serum electrolytes, VO2 Max [14]. The most commonly used heat strain indicators in previous studies are core body temperature, resting heart rate, working heart rate, recovery heart rate and sweat rate. These are done in non invasive manner, so it is easy to perform in field based study. Other parameters such as urine specific gravity, serum electrolytes, creatinine, Vo2 max though reliable but could not be used in the field based study due to the constraints faced in working environment. In fact, these parameters were used in experimental set up study rather than actual field based study. Methods to measure these parameters vary in different study. The most commonly used instrument to measure the core body temperature is through tympanic thermometer as tympanic temperature is the reliable, convenient and most easily accessible site to measure core body temperature (**Figure 2**). Polar heart rate monitor was used to measure the different heart rate in working environment as it is capable of recording continuous heart rate (**Figure 3**). Sweat rate was measured by using the body weight and fluid intake and output of the worker during the working period. The most commonly preferred method to measure the heat strain indicators is to check the pre exposure and post exposure values of these parameters as it can be compared with the standard values given by ACGIH, OSHA etc.

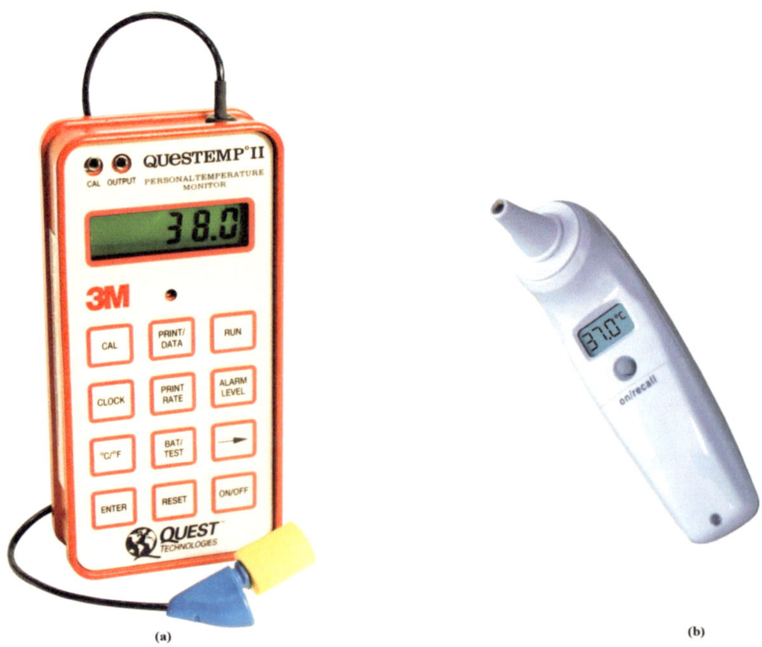

Figure 2.
Tympanic thermometer: (a) quest temp personal monitor, (b) Infrared tympanic thermometer.

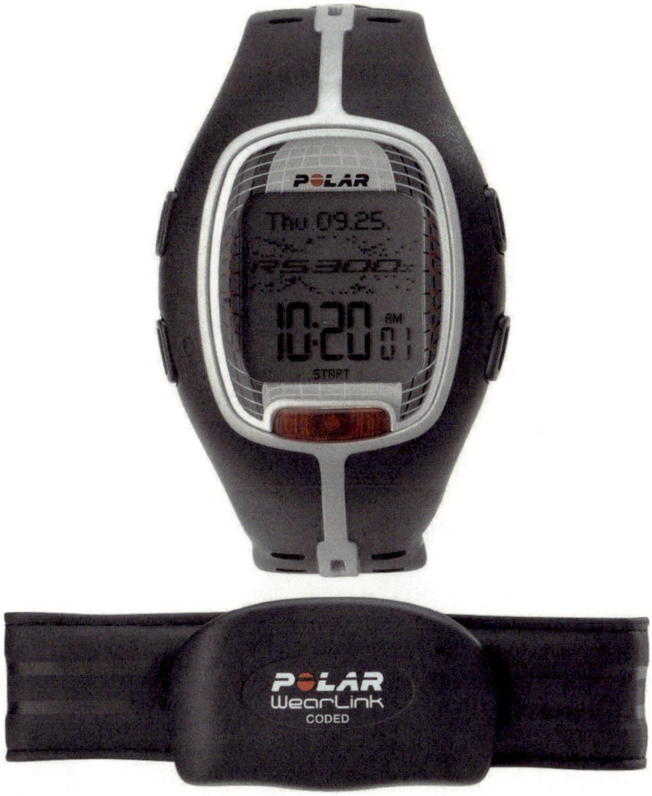

Figure 3.
Polar heart rate monitor.

5. Who is at risk?

Elderly people above 50 years, pregnant women, workers with other co morbid conditions are at increased risk of developing heat related illness. Most of the functions of the human organs are dependent on the temperature and pH. So if there is alteration in any of these two, then it will definitely have impact on other functions of human body. Workers with history of diabetes mellitus, hypertension, and thyroid disorder are at increased risk as it will cause extra burden to the various organs while working in hot environment. Workers at risk of heat stress include outdoor workers such as agriculture, brick industry, construction and indoor occupation such as firefighters, bakery workers, miners, boiler room workers, factory workers. The major reason that working people belongs to vulnerable group is because of internal heat produced when muscles are used during work [14]. Some people tend to keep working beyond the safe limit for heat exposure because of their need to complete work tasks during a particular period or their need to maintain work output to get paid [24]. During prolonged work periods in the heat, the high sweat rates leads to progressive dehydration. It has been well documented that losses of fluids through sweating can lead to dehydration which has a detrimental effect on productivity.

6. Health hazards due to heat stress exposure

When the air temperature or humidity rises above the optimal ranges for comfort, can leads to health impacts [14]. The initial effects are subjective in nature, they often relate to how you feel. Exposure to more heat stress for a longer duration can cause health problems which impair workers' ability to execute the task and may cause adverse health effects [10]. The body temperature increases because of internal heat production during muscular activity in work place. If the ambient temperature is more than the body temperature, then the heat loss from the body will be minimized by conduction, convection, radiation. As a result the core body temperature will keep increasing and may result in heat related illness such as heat rash, heat syncope, heat exhaustion, heat stroke. The heart rate also increases to pump more blood through skin so that excess heat can be lost to the environment through sweating [14]. These changes will cause additional load on the body. Changes in blood flow and excessive sweating will lead to decrease in person's ability to do physical and mental work [8]. When the environmental temperature rises above 30°C, it may interfere with the performance of mental tasks [14]. The occupational heat stress can affect the workers health either directly or indirectly. The direct health impacts include the heat related illness such as heat rash, heat syncope, heat edema, heat exhaustion and heat stroke [6, 14]. The indirect health impacts include physical and mental stress, hypertension, diabetes mellitus and chronic kidney disease.

Heat rashes are the red spots on the skin which cause a prickling sensation during heat exposure. Heat edema is swelling which generally occurs among people who are not acclimatized to working in hot conditions. Heat cramps are sharp pains in the muscles that may occur as a result of salt imbalance resulting from the failure to replace salt lost due to sweating. Heat exhaustion is caused by excessive loss of body water and salt through excessive sweating. Heat syncope is heat-induced giddiness and fainting because of insufficient flow of blood to the brain while a person is standing which is caused by the loss of body fluids through sweating. Heat stroke is the most serious types of heat illnesses. The body temperature often increases more than 41°C.

7. Status of research in occupational heat stress

The environmental temperature increases day by day to due to the ongoing climate change that is occurring in various part of the world. Deforestation, urban heat island effect, Modernization process, increase in number of industries cause a rise in ambient temperature level, which also has impacts on workers health. Studies pertaining to heat stress across the globe are carried by researchers and they have found that exposure to excessive heat in work place has impacts on workers health and productivity.

Studies in occupational heat stress in India are limited because of the following challenges and constraints [25].

a. Permission from Industries to collect data and to publish it

b. Organized vs. Unorganized sector

c. Improper record/documentation of heat/any occupational disease by the employer or worker

d. Study Design

e. Assessment of health parameters

Specific heat wave events in the Northern hemisphere have been associated with marked short term increases in mortality, with reported excess mortality ranging from 4–142% [4]. It is estimated that in 2003, up to 70,000 additional deaths occurred over the summer months in Western Europe as a consequence of severe heat waves [26]. An estimated 560 extra deaths were observed during the three heat waves of 2002 in Russia. Lag times of just a few days have been observed between the onset of a heat wave and the rise in mortality, suggesting that people succumb quickly to the effects of extreme heat. Some of the deaths occurring in heat waves are due to exacerbation of preexisting illnesses particularly cardiovascular and respiratory diseases, and diseases of the nervous system [27]. Mortality associated with heat waves has been reported to be greatest in city areas, in conjunction with observed high night-time minimum temperatures, high levels of air pollution, and poor housing conditions. Few studies have investigated the effects of extreme hot weather on population morbidity. Hospital admissions have been observed to increase during heat waves. However studies have revealed discrepancies between the impact of heat waves on morbidity and mortality, in terms of magnitude, cause, and age group [28]. Reports of a lesser impact of heat waves on hospital admissions than on mortality may indicate that people die quickly during heat waves before they are able to reach hospital or be noticed by others. Studies of patients admitted to hospitals during heat waves for treatment of heatstroke have shown this illness to be associated with an outcome. The risk of heat stroke among working people is well known and explained by the limits of human physiological adaptability [14]. Significant number of working people dies due to heat stroke even in high income countries as described in a study of agricultural workers in the USA. A substantial amount of body water may be lost as sweat, including loss of fluid through respiration, gastrointestinal tract as well as kidney. Increased dehydration disturbs the homeostasis of the body, leading to decreased skin blood flow, elevated core body temperature, decreased sweat rate leading to impaired to tolerance to work resulting in increased risks of heat injuries. Continuous exposure to excessive heat may cause profound increase in heart rate which may lead to sympatho - vagal imbalance if not treated appropriately [20]. Heart rate is useful in evaluating the exertion required by physical labour in working conditions [22]. Trainings including acclimatization may be useful in maintaining the core body temperature and heart rate within normal range among workers exposed to excessive heat [17]. A wide range of clinical observations & measurements have been used to indicate heat strain, ranging from perception of workers to hospitalization due to heat stroke. > 20% of people are being estimated to have health impacts of heat stress, ranging from skin rash to heat stroke. About 28% of workers were at risk of health impairment due to high heat exposure at work place [29]. There was a noticeable disconnect between worker's perceptions and their ability to perform task [30]. Most of these studies were done in experimental set up which cannot be considered as a standard protocol for studies in field/industry. Some of the examples include rectal temperature, capsule method for core body temperature, nude body weight measurement, etc. Apart from heat, many confounding factors also play a role in health impacts. With all this issues, it is important to identify globally acceptable heat strain parameters and methods. Such methods can be used as relevant indicators locally by the health professionals to develop health surveillance and prevention programs for workers to protect the workers health. There are only few studies done in India about Occupational heat stress and its health impacts and no studies conducted on assessment of heat stress and its physiological responses in this geographical location. So it is very essential to do more studies in India to document the health impacts of heat stress.

8. Prevention and control

Prevention is better than cure. It will be ideal for each worker to follow certain preventive measures to reduce the health impacts due to heat stress. The prevention methods may vary with different occupational sectors. The occupational sectors can broadly be classified in to outdoor (Unorganized) and indoor sector (organized). Adequate rest, following work rest cycle, providing adequate fluid during work time can be followed as a preventive measure in outdoor sector. Along with these measures, engineering intervention such as providing fan, coolers, PPE can also be followed in indoor sectors as prevention and control measures. Health education about the heat stress and its health impacts will greatly help to reduce the burden of the disease [6].

- Educating the management and administrative members to provide training to the workers regarding heat strain at the time of employment
- Health education is very important for the workers.
- Advised workers to consult doctor if any health problem is noticed by the worker
- Periodic health assessment of the workers (health surveillance)
- Suggestions for engineering intervention such as proper ventilation, exhaust, work rest cycle can be given to the management

9. Adaptive measures

Heat exposure levels can be lowered by use of certain control measures such as engineering intervention (Proving fan, coolers), personal protective equipments, proper ventilation, adequate rest, following work rest cycle as per ACGIH guidelines, providing adequate fluid to prevent dehydration, periodic medical checkup, etc. Special attention should be provided to aged workers and also to workers with significant medical illness. Health education to workers regarding heat related illness and ways to prevent it can help in reducing the morbidity. Studies of this kind using mapping can help in detecting the vulnerable areas inside the industry and also can protect the workers health. All workers should be made aware of the heat levels in all the areas inside the industry and should be instructed to take all precautionary measures while working in high heat generating areas. Engineering controls like by providing fan, adequate ventilation in working environment and by following work rest cycle as per ACGIH guidelines can protect the workers health. These recommendations could help the workers to protect their health from heat related illness.

10. Conclusion

Occupational heat stress will cause potential negative health with wellbeing outcome. The industries (Management) and the workers should be educated about the health impacts of occupational heat stress. Proper measures should be laid down to prevent the heat related illness which can be helpful to reduce the morbidity and mortality that may indirectly improve the community economy.

Author details

Krishnan Srinivasan*, Smisha Mohan and Jeneth Berlin Raj T
Department of Physiology, Mahatma Gandhi Medical College and Research Institute, Sri Balaji Vidyapeeth, Puducherry, India

*Address all correspondence to: drkrish10@gmail.com

References

[1] American Conference of Governmental Industrial Hygienists (ACGIH). Threshold Limits Value for Chemical Substances and Physical Agents &Biological Exposure Indices. Cincinnati, OH, USA, 2010; 206-215.

[2] Kjellstrom T, Butler AJ, Lucas RM, Bonita R. Public health impact of global heating due to climate change: potential effects on chronic non-communicable diseases. Int J Public Health .2010; 55: 97-103.

[3] Dash S. K, Kjellstrom T. Workplace heat stress in the context of rising temperature in India. Current Science. 2011; 101 (4): 496-503.

[4] IPCC Climate Change: Synthesis Report. Contribution of Working Groups I, II and III to the Fourth Assessment Report of the Inter-governmental Panel on Climate Change. 2007.

[5] CDC - Heat Stress - NIOSH Workplace Safety and Health Topic". www.cdc.gov. Retrieved 2016-04-15.

[6] NIOSH Criteria for a Recommended Standard: Occupational Exposure to Heat and Hot Environments". 2016. doi:10.26616/NIOSHPUB2016106.

[7] Rebekah A I Lucas, Yoram Epstein, Tord Kjellstrom. Excessive occupational heat exposure: a significant ergonomic challenge and health risk for current and future workers. Extreme Physiology & Medicine. 2014; 3(14). 71-78.

[8] Hancock PA, Vasmatzidis I. Effects of heat stress on cognitive performance: the current state of knowledge. Int J Hyperthermia. 2003; 19:355-372.

[9] Krishnamurthy M, Paramesh Ramalingam, Kumaravel Perumal, Latha Perumal Kamalakannan, Jeremiah Chinnadurai, Rekha Shanmugam, Krishnan Srinivasan, Vidhya Venugopal. Occupational heat stress impacts on health and productivity in a steel industry in southern India. Safety and Health at Work. 2017; 8(1):99-104.

[10] Rodahl. Occupational Health Conditions in Extreme Environments. Ann Occup Hyg. 2003; 47 (3): 241-252.

[11] Vinod Joon, Vaishali Jaiswal. Impact of climate change on human health in India: an overview. Health and Population - Perspectives and Issues.2012; 35(1):11-22.

[12] Nag PK, Nag A. Shiftwork in the hot environment. J. Hum. Ergol. 2001; 30: 161-166.

[13] Vidhya Venugopal, Jeremiah S. Chinnadurai , Rebekah A. I. Lucas, Tord Kjellstrom. Occupational heat stress profiles in selected workplaces in India. Int. J. Environ. Res. Public Health. 2016; 13: 89-95.

[14] Parsons KC. Human Thermal Environments: The Effects of Hot, Moderate and Cold Temperatures on Human Health, Comfort and Performance, 2nd ed.; Taylor & Francis: London, UK, 2003.

[15] Kelly GS. Body temperature variability (Part 2): masking influences of body temperature variability and a review of body temperature variability in disease. Altern Med Rev. 2007; 12 (1): 49-62.

[16] RS Bridger. Introduction to Ergonomics. 2nd ed. Taylor & Francis, London; 2003.

[17] Peter Bröde, Schütte Martin Kampmann, Bernhard Griefahn Barbara. Heat acclimation and its relation to resting core temperature and heart rate. Occupational Ergonomics. 2009; 8(4): 185-193.

[18] Mackowiak P A, S S Wasserman, M M Levine. A critical appraisal of 98.6 degrees F, the upper limit of the normal body temperature, and other legacies of Carl Reinhold August Wunderlich. JAMA.1992; 268 (12): 1578-1580.

[19] Parsons K. Heat stress standard ISO 7243 and its global application. Ind Health. 2006; 44: 368-379.

[20] Habibollah Dehghan, Seyed Bagher Mortazavi, Mohammad Javad Jafari. The evaluation of heat stress through monitoring environmental factors and Physiological responses in melting and casting industries workers. Int J Env Health Eng. 2012; 1(2): 1-5.

[21] Graham P Bates, Schneider J. Hydration status and physiological workload of UAE construction workers: A prospective longitudinal observational study. Journal of Occupational Medicine and Toxicology. 2008; 3(1): 24-30.

[22] Yamamoto S, Iwamoto M, Inoue M, Harada N. Evaluation of the effect of heat exposure on the autonomic nervous system by heart rate variability and urinary catecholamines. J Occup Health. 2007; 4 (9): 199-204.

[23] Aliasghar Farshad, Saideh Montazer, Mohammad Reza Monazzam, Meysam Eyvazlou, Roksana Mirkazemi. Heat stress level among construction workers. Iranian J Publ Health. 2014; 43 (4): 492-498.

[24] Kjellstrom T, Lemke B, Otto M. Mapping occupational heat exposure and effects in South-East Asia: ongoing time trends 1980-2011 and future estimates to 2050. Ind Health. 2013; 51(1):56-67.

[25] Srinivasan K, Maruthy KN, Venugopal V, Ramaswamy P. Research in occupational heat stress in India: Challenges and opportunities. Indian J Occup Environ Med. 2017; 20: 73-78

[26] Karin Lundgren, Kalev Kuklane, Chuansi Gao, Ingvar Holmér. Effect of heat stress in working population when facing a climate change. Ind Health. 2013; 51:3-15

[27] Allyson S Howe, Barry P Boden. Heat-related illness in athletes. The American Journal of Sports Medicine. 2007; 35(8): 1384-1395.

[28] Rupa Basu, Jonathan M. Samet. Relation between elevated ambient temperature and mortality: A review of the epidemiologic evidence. Epidemiologic Reviews. 2002; 24(2): 190-202.

[29] Ramalingam Ayyappan, Sambandam Sankar, Paramasivan Rajkumar and Kalpana Balakrishnan. Work-related heat stress concerns in automotive industries: a case study from Chennai, India. Glob Health Action. 2009; DOI: 10.3402/gha.v2i0.2060

[30] Kalpana Balakrishnan, Ayyappan Ramalingam, Venkatesan Dasu, Jeremiah Chinnadurai Stephen, Mohan Raj Sivaperumal, Deepan Kumarasamy, Krishnendu Mukhopadhyay, Santu Ghosh and Sankar Sambandam. Case studies on heat stress related perceptions in different industrial sectors in southern India. Glob Health Action. 2010; 3: 5635 - DOI: 10.3402/gha. v3i0.5635

Chapter 11

Managing Inter-Organizational Knowledge Sharing: Integrating Macro, Meso and Micro Level Analysis

Chiraz Guedda

Abstract

Numerous studies focus on the increasing role that cooperation plays on knowledge creation and the importance of knowledge diversity. However, in dealing with different background, culture, process, and knowledge throughout collaborative project, organizations must improve their practices to access, share and create knowledge. This paper aims at highlighting the complexity of interfirm collaborative projects while analyzing how different factors bolster knowledge sharing between partners depend on project phases. This work supports literature on interactionist approaches and project management to analyze these concepts of collaboration and knowledge sharing. Based on case study of an aerospace cluster, the findings highlight the factors that may enhances the effectiveness of knowledge sharing depend on project phases. We conclude by identifying further conceptual research and implication for research and practice.

Keywords: collaboration, ecosystem, knowledge sharing, project

1. Introduction

In today economy's, knowledge becomes more and more critical for organizational survival and competitiveness. Both researchers and practitioners have emphasized the need to develop, refine and access to knowledge to ensure the innovative capacity of organizations [1, 2] and hence their competitiveness. In this context, mainstream literature on knowledge management considers that process which leads to knowledge creation and innovation requires to cooperate with actors inside and across the boundaries of organizations. The success of certain innovative regions such as Silicon Valley and Route 128 of Boston, which argue that these industrial location models or clusters are a source of economic progress for the local communities' regions and consequently the nations, sheds light on the localized nature of innovation. In fact, the clusters are seen as the driver to the development of knowledge economies based around innovation [3–5]. In this way, innovation is seen more and more as a social, collective and localized process.

The literature on clusters provides useful insights that explain the factors that enhance knowledge creation and innovation within the cluster. Most of these research analyses the role of proximities in facilitating the collaboration and knowledge sharing. However, despite the widespread expansion of research on concepts of cluster, recent studies emphasize the current analytical shortcomings and the failure of conceptualizing innovation in contemporary societies [6], the lack of understanding the dynamics of collaboration within the cluster [7–9], and the little known in the explanation of the link between knowledge ties and proximity within the cluster [10]. As cluster enhances innovation by facilitating knowledge creation, the aim of this research is to shed light in the factors that bolster knowledge sharing between partners. To do so, we draw from research on cluster and knowledge management to analysis the factors that enhance and impeded the interorganizational knowledge sharing. In the sections that follow, we first review research on collaboration, cluster and knowledge sharing highlighting the factors that foster or impede the interorganizational knowledge sharing within a cluster. Section 2 explains the methodological framework used for this research and in the final section we summarize the findings as well as future research directions.

2. Literature review

2.1 Inter-organizational collaboration and ecosystem

Business today is based on networks and collaboration within and between organizations. As, knowledge is dispersed among different actors and organizations [11, 12] a most relevant motivation of organizations is the access to new ideas and complementary knowledge resources [13, 14]. In fact, knowledge diversity resulting of these collaborations enhance innovation as it is seen to expand the range of ideas that individual can use. Increasingly, literature on innovation considers industrial clusters [15, 16], national system of innovation [5], business ecosystem [17] and ecosystem of innovation [18–20] as territorial systems that facilitates and drive collaboration. Whatever name they are given, these concepts are widely analyzed to better understand the nature of relation between space industry and innovation [6]. For both researchers and practitioners, much of this intense interest is driven by the recognition that co-location allows the generation of a learning process, following the externalities of knowledge generated by geographical proximity, thus leading to innovation [15, 21, 22]. Mostly based on the success of certain highly innovative regions such as Silicon Valley and Route 128 of Boston, the unanimity about the virtues of these forms of territorial agglomeration has been reinforced. Local production system is here referred to under the generic term of «ecosystem» which is defined as *« an economic community supported by a foundation of interacting organizations and individuals-the organisms of the business world. This economic community produces goods and services of value to customers, who are themselves members of the ecosystem» ([17]*:26). As Moore [17] states, the ecosystem refers primarily to notions of interdependence, leadership, and coevolution around innovative ideas.

More and more, innovation is seen as a collective action, which involves many different actors operating in a cluster context [23]. Furthermore, cluster enhances interorganizational relationship among the actors by facilitating networking and socialization through the geographic proximity [24, 25]. This socialization, facilitated by the possibility of frequent face-to-face contacts, helps foster knowledge exchange by building trust [26, 27]. As Cohendet et al. [28] argued, what are matters in the socio-economic approach of networks is the quality of the relationship between firms rather than the quality of the transaction. This social dimension's interest in the relationship between the partners has led to more and more in-depth research on the notion of social proximity. As it is increasingly recognized that the knowledge economy is a relational economy [29], much of research on networks and collaboration [30, 31] knowledge management [26] has stressed the benefit of social proximity to facilitate collaboration and knowledge sharing. As suggested by the literature of sociology [32], social proximity fosters trust and builds a mutual commitment and consequently facilitates collaboration and interactive learning. In other words, it is often highlighted that the network partners may generate new solutions by joint-problem solving arrangements facilitated by ties embedded in the network [31]. As Boschma et al. [33] and Boschma [34] explain, an innovative performance at the firm follows an inverted «U» relationship between embeddedness and firm's innovative performance. Boschma [34] uses the embededness literature [32, 35] to define social proximity as a micro level' socially embedded relationships that includes trust based on friendship, kinship, and experience. This social proximity fosters the interactive learning by reducing the risk of opportunistic behavior and facilitating the sharing of tacit knowledge [26], which requires frequent interactions. However, Boschma [34] argue that as well as too much social distance, too much social proximity may be harmful for learning and innovation as it could lead to a closed community and consequently impedes innovation by limiting the access to the innovative ideas and diversity.

2.2 Ecosystem and knowledge sharing

Knowledge creation and innovation processes have become increasingly complex due to a wide variety of sources of knowledge and the growing need for collaboration [7, 36]. The main purpose of theses collaboration is to maintain a sustainable advantage [37] by creating and sharing knowledge. Corno et al. [38] present three levels of knowledge transfer. The level of «initiation» that allows the sharing of explicit knowledge, the «encounter» level in which the actors seek to understand the tacit knowledge of their partners, to convert them into explicit knowledge, to integrate and to use them, and the level of «intimacy», in which the interaction between partners becomes deeper and characterizes a more developed level of cooperation between them. In this phase, the partners exchange their tacit knowledge by sharing their experiences, exchanging their culture and adopting a common language.

Different factors can influence the success of knowledge sharing. The overview of the literature highlights these main factors in [18] the characteristics of the units involved in the sense of their motivation and their cognitive and absorption capacity [19, 39–42] the attributes of knowledge [11, 39, 40, 42, 43] the relationships between partners [7, 38, 39, 42] the organizational context [41, 44] and [39] the network properties [45]. However, most of these researches examine the factors facilitating the knowledge transfer and sharing by using one level of analysis such individual or team or organization.

The present qualitative interpretative research seek to better understand inter-organizational knowledge sharing process. It adopts an interactionist approach as stipulated by Strauss [46] is divided into three main elements: [18] the society as a collective production resulting from the interaction between different actors [19] the competences the knowledge and the rules are essentially elaborated in inter-subjective relations that evolve over time and [11] the human being must be seen as an active, reflective and creative being. The review of literature shows that the knowledge sharing between ecosystem partners needs a deeper understanding of the factors and determinants that enhance the knowledge sharing and how that affect it. Little is known about the determinants of successful knowledge sharing [47]. The present qualitative research seeks to better understand interorganizational knowledge sharing process between interorganizational projects partners by answering those two main questions: what are the factors that bolster knowledge sharing between partners? How these factors emerge during the collaborative project?

3. Research methodology

3.1 Case study

This research studies knowledge sharing between collaborative project partners within an innovative ecosystem. As the Quebecer aerospace ecosystem is an innovative ecosystem, it provides an interesting case for understanding collaborative projects and knowledge sharing processes. Our case of study is the projects of the Consortium for Research and Innovation in Aerospace in Quebec (CRIAQ). The Consortium for Research and Innovation in Aerospace in Quebec (CRIAQ) is a non-profit organization (NPO) created in 2002 with the financial support of the Quebec government. Including companies of all size, academics and research centres as actors, CRIAQ aims to improve the collective knowledge base in the aerospace industry and to increase its competitiveness. CRIAQ operates in a network based on logic of open innovation and promotes collaboration between specialists from industry and researchers to identify and implement projects that meet industry requirements. His mission is to stimulate the ecosystem innovation by increasing collaborative projects and to enhance the skills and knowledge of aerospace actors. For CRIAQ projects, the funding structure determines the allocation of leadership within the team. Indeed, since the 50% of funding comes from NSERC (Natural Sciences and Engineering Research Council), it was agreed that leadership should be attributed to the university partner. As conceived by Etzkowitz and Leydesdroff [48], the CRIAQ model is strongly built on the interrelationship and interdependence between three spheres: state, industry and university and provides three analysis level: macro, meso and micro.

3.2 Level of analysis

Our objective is to understand the dynamics of knowledge sharing between the partners of the aeronautical sector. Thus, the unit of analysis focuses on individual involved in collaborative projects. However, we adopt a systemic analysis that includes the micro (individual), meso (organization) and macro (ecosystem) level.

3.3 Data collection

To collect data, we used semi-structured in-depth interview and documentation nevertheless, our main source of data collection is the semi-structured in-depth interview. The documentation as second source of data collection were collected through forum and steering committee records allows us to provide as much information as possible on the subject and field of our study, but also to triangulate our data sources. Regular follow-up interviews, secondary data analysis (internal documents), and corroboration activities were conducted to ensure that our findings match interviewees' view of reality. The triangulation of different data sources (interviews and documentation) makes it possible to identify converging lines, to corroborate information from other data sources [49]. As Eisenhardt [50] suggested, the data collection process was stopped when the interviews brought little or no more new information.

3.4 Sampling

As suggested by Eisenhardt [50] and Eisenhardt and Graebner [51], we conducted a theoretical sample by choosing cases that present a theoretical contribution for our study. As our sample is composed of 5 sub-samples: [18] main contractors [19] integrators and Tier One suppliers [11] governmental and consortia organizations [7] universities and research centers and [39] SMEs, for the semi-structured interviews we sought theoretical saturation [50] in each category of respondents. This implies that we did not seek an equal number of interviews between the 5 subsamples. **Table 1** presents the respondent's profiles and the numbers of interviews conducted.

In addition to academics, respondents hold the positions of: President, Vice President (Technology and Innovation), Vice President (R&D), General Manager, Project Director, Technical Director, R&D Director, Head of Department. These respondents are directly involved in CRIAQ projects at the decision-making and/or operational level. These different positions of informants involved in collaborative CRIAQ projects allows us to better understand the motivations of the partners, the context of the projects (decision making process to collaborate) which allows us a deeper analysis of the determinants that bolster the knowledge sharing between partners.

However, two main criteria were important for the constitution of the sampling:

1. The sampling must include respondents belonging to each aeronautic ecosystem actors: major contractors, equipment manufacturers and SMEs, universities and research centers, public actors (ministries), and research consortia and another public-private organization involved in the aeronautical ecosystem and in connection with research consortia.

2. The informant must be involved inclusively in (i) at least one completed CRIAQ project and (ii) another collaborative internal projects to their respective organizations. By the first element, which is at least one CRIAQ project, we sought to guarantee more richness of data through the experience of the respondent throughout all the CRIAQ projects phases. Thus, we excluded from our data analysis two cases of respondents who participated only in a CRIAQ project which is in progress, because we judged that the interviews were not sufficiently rich since the respondents did not necessarily have a complete vision of the project. Our objective is to understand the dynamic of knowledge sharing between partners in the aeronautical sector, it is therefore implicit that the respondents must have experienced all the phases of the collaborative project. However, without carrying out a formal comparative analysis between the two types of projects (internal and CRIAQ projects) in our analysis, for the second element, which is being involved in other collaborative projects internal to the organization, this will also allow us a deeper understanding of the dynamic of collaboration of the organization. This will essentially allow us to understand the impact of the two levels: meso and macro.

3.5 Semi structured interviews

We conducted 52 semi-structured one -on- one interviews with various aerospace industry stakeholders involved in CRIAQ's projects including academics (professors), industrials and government institutions. The interview lasted approximately between 30 to 80 minutes and were conducted over an 11 months period. The interview process was based on an interview guide. Taking into account the flexible attitude adopted during interviews, this interview guide is more of an interview support and not a static interview guide and sets out the topics that should be covered during the interview. It is important to note that the terminology used in the interview guide is not the same as that used in the conceptual

Types of organizations	Number of interviews
Main contractors	15
SME	10
OEMs, Integrators and MROs- Tier One Suppliers	8
Governmental organizations and consortia	7
Universities and research centers	12
Total	52

Table 1.
The study respondent's profiles.

framework. This difference is explained by the concern of clarity which requires the use of terms understandable by the respondents and which are part of their reference scheme [52]. A first version of the guide has been served as a pre-test for our interview guide and aims to validate final interview guide. Two main versions of the interview guide were developed: a version (A) addressed to academics and industry and a version (B) addressed to government actors and consortia. These two versions take into account the particularities of the partner actors in collaborative projects and differ slightly and mainly in terms of the theme dealing with the progress of the project and knowledge management. Indeed, government actors and those belonging to the sub-sample of consortia do not actively participate in all project phases (especially in the execution phase) but are more involved in the initiation and set up phases some questions then differ from those asked of industrial and university partners. The interview guide consists of two parts. The first part involved general questions about the informants' background, their experience in collaborative projects. The second section focused on the main purpose of the study which is the determinants of knowledge sharing. The purpose of this section is to collect the information, experiences thoughts and interpretations of respondents regarding the progress of the collaborative's projects and its outcomes in terms of knowledge sharing. In addition, in this interview section, we often encouraged and asked respondents to provide us with concrete examples in order to enrich our data with real-life experiences.

3.6 Data analysis

The data analysis strategy adopted in our study follows the assumptions of the grounded theory. This strategy involves "the systematic comparison of small units of data (incidents) and the gradual construction of a system of" categories "that describe the phenomena being observed" [53]. The data has been condensed, structured and analysed. The data analysis followed the three types of coding of the grounded theory described by Corbin and Strauss [54], Corley and Gioia [55] and Charmaz [56]: open coding, axial coding and selective coding (or theoretical coding). To do so, we conducted line-by -line analysis of every quote to identify common ideas [57]. Through an iterative process, we defined a sub-category, and we established the link between the various categories by questioning causes, how, where and when [58]. Linking these categories allows us to assemble into higher order themes ([55]: 183). Thus, by establishing the relationships between categories and subcategories and integrating the concepts around the central themes, we can provide better explanations of the dynamic of knowledge sharing between collaborative project partners. The analysis is summarized in Appendix 1.

4. Results

The purpose of this research was to better understand the factors driving the knowledge sharing in the context of inter-organizational collaboration. This work aims at analyzing how different determinants bolster the knowledge sharing process between partners. Based on the results of our primary data, these determinants depend on projects' phases as well as analysis level (macro, meso and micro). The research finding shows that the role of social proximity played an important role in the initiation project' phases, especially by fostering collaboration, but throughout the project its apport is controverted. As well, during this phase, the macro level, via the quasi- governmental institutions, helped fostering collaboration and knowledge sharing between aerospace partners. The team dynamic and the organization culture are more determinants in the set-up and execution project' phases while the role of macro level actors is less important.

4.1 Knowledge sharing and project' phases

We deemed it appropriate to present the determinants and issues that influence collaboration between partners according to the phases in which they emerge. This choice is strongly influenced by the primary data which led us to classify the categories of determinants according to the project phases. These different phases are project initiation phase, project setup phase and the project execution phase. The determinants that influence knowledge sharing are related to three levels: micro, meso and macro. The purpose of this research was to better understand the underlying factors driving the knowledge sharing in the context of inter-organizational collaboration. The research finding shows that the role of social proximity in fostering collaboration is controverted. Despite the importance of the social proximity in collaboration, our results highlight that the outcomes of this collaboration, in term of success of collaboration and knowledge sharing, are questionable. In fact, our results reveal how the critical is the role that institutions play in facilitating collaboration among actors and creating an enabling environment for co-innovation. However, our results have also shown that despite the willingness and efforts of public actors to stimulate the process of co-innovation between actors, this objective does not seem to be easily achievable. The success of collaborative activity now depends on other determinants of individual and organizational nature, depending on the progress of the project.

4.1.1 The initiation project phase: the role of micro and macro level

The initiation project' phases highlight the importance of the micro and macro level in the knowledge sharing process. It was particularly noticeable that informants argued that the macro level provides a great condition fostering knowledge sharing and collaboration. For example, the CRIAQ' forum, organized every two years, present the opportunity for the aerospace actors to openly display their issues and their research needs. The objective of those forum is to help organisations and academics to enhance their skills and develop their knowledge by sharing, exploring a new problematic. At this level, it is important to specify that the principal mission of CRIAQ is to bolster collaboration which is leads to knowledge sharing. However, some informants felt that, despite the role of CRIAQ fostering collaboration, the social capital is the most determinant element at this phase.

4.1.1.1 Social proximity: the challenge

Participants' statements such as «it's because I have good relation», «he's a nice guy», «we look at affinities», «the research is between friends» and «if the chemistry is not there it does not work!» have been widely given as an answer to explain their choice of projects partners. Facilitated by the geographic proximity, the social proximity is shown as a foster for the emergence of collaborative project and an important determinant for the knowledge sharing process. According to our results, social capital is dependent on past experiences, friendship and affinities between actors. Those relationships are consolidated by the trust that people develop among themselves through their previous experiences and their evolution over time. Specifically, partners develop their trust in each other based on knowledge, trustworthiness and friendship. This is reflected in the comments of one of our respondents: «we create a certain trust between the players through the relationship» and «the social aspect is an important element that I had underestimated! That's where trust comes in! ». However, curiously, despite the importance of social proximity during the initiation phase of the project, our results throughout the progress of project, the social proximity does not play an important role. Social proximity facilitates the emergence of collaborative project, but it does not always mean it that lead to collaboration none achieve knowledge sharing.

4.1.2 The set-up' project phase: the role of meso level

The set-up project' phases highlight the importance of meso level in the knowledge sharing process. According to most of informants, the team project partners and the organisation' implication played an important role to facilitate the knowledge sharing process during the set-up projects phases.

4.1.2.1 Institutional orientation

The research results highlight the crucial role of institutional orientation of the firm and how it affects the goal of collaborative project and consequently the knowledge sharing process. Indeed, for most of our informants the involvement of the industrial firm in the CRIAQ project is seen rather as a response to a social mission, political pressure and a need for visibility. It is therefore not surprising that the organization' interest in the CRIAQ project is sometimes low and questionable. Consequently, it is obvious that the availability of team members on these projects is compromised. One of informants explained: *«So it limits the frequency of meetings, the availability of industrial very much limits the frequency of meetings ... Then if people are not available, also sometimes it puts frustrations when we want to settle things and then there is no availability»*. The lack of availability affects deeply the purpose of collaboration and knowledge sharing process between partners. As the team partners do not have the availability needed to the project progress, they do not necessarily absorb and integrate in time the information and new knowledge generated by the project. In these cases, the challenge is to take advantage of this information before it becomes obsolete. This informant summarized this issue: *«So often, we will absorb the information in detail a few years later. Because when the project starts, we do not have the resources, we do not have the right resources. We follow the project, but how can I say.. with a certain distance, we are not equipped, and we do not do it from day to day»*. However, the lack of project interest showed two different explanations from informant. In one hand, informants stated that the "bottom up" approach of these collaborative project does not lead necessarily to knowledge sharing process and in other hand, others informant explained that this lack in the interest in the project is a consequence of the absence of some individual's determinants such as communication, leaderships, insufficient skills in project management.

4.1.3 The execution' project phase: the role of micro level

According to informants, the most important determinant to foster knowledge sharing process is leadership. As stated earlier, social proximity and affinities are just not enough to bolster knowledge sharing process. Sometimes, with disappointment some of informants explained that most of CRIAQ projects are based on social proximity to choose team projects partners. However, despite this social proximity, informants argued that tension and disappointment are experienced during most of CRIAQ project especially during the execution phases the project when the role of leader is much needed. It is worth noting that based on the rules of CRIAQ project, the academic partner should take the lead of project. Most of informants explained that the lack of «strong leader» described as problematic and lead to frustration and loss of project interest. Some respondents explain: «there are several universities and research center and they do not necessarily communicate, it's the job of academic lead normally, it's hard to promote these communications!», «Yes it slows down our involvement in CRIAQ projects definitely. Yes definitely! It's a matter of credibility...We say it starts today, but we will start in a year!». However, our results show that the leadership issues is related to misunderstanding of the reality of each other's partners. For the academic's partners, it is not lack of "strong leader" that impact the execution of project but the misunderstanding of industrials partners of the academic' challenge to build the research team. One of academic informants explained: "Sometimes that's why we can't deliver or start on time because of student recruitment, for some projects we cannot recruit international student, and because of the ability of manufacturers to bring out data internally and communicate it to us... They ask us the impossible". On the whole, the research results show the challenge that face the partners of interorganizational collaborative project especially between academics and industrials partners. For the academic' partners the feeling of misunderstanding of their realities and the challenges they faced is widely raised. In fact, despite the collaborative aspect of these project, this divide on the way how to perceive partners 'reality and challenge makes the knowledge sharing process not easy to achieve.

5. Discussion

The purpose of this paper was to gain an in depth understanding the factors that impede and foster the inter-organizational knowledge sharing within a collaborative project. The results highlight how social proximity, which is considerate as a facilitator to collaboration and interactive learning, is needed to initiate the collaborative project but neither fosters collaboration nor facilitates the knowledge sharing process in a lack of other factors. Our finding suggests that throughout the project' progress, the lack of leadership and interest in the project tracked a failure to achieve a knowledge sharing between partners. Indeed, open innovation requires leadership [59]. Overall, more specifically, our results highlighted the existence of deep tensions and frustrations between the collaborative project' partners especially between academia and industry. As explained by open innovation and ecosystem research, the need of complementary knowledge is more and more needed through a cross-boundary collaborations. These interorganizational collaboration implies partners with different background and culture working interdependently across disciplines arises challenges and makes knowledge sharing between partners more complex.

5.1 Interorganizational knowledge sharing challenge

Despite the complementarities between the aeronautic ecosystem partners and the need of a new knowledge, this study shows a challenging relation between two important actors: the industrials and the academics. In fact, universities have become a major knowledge creator in many countries [60]. Our finding shows a challenging collaboration between the academics and industries.

5.2 Academics-industrial: complementarities with two languages

Innovation is needed in today's challenging environment which dynamism and managing uncertainty is required [61]. Open innovation which is "a paradigm that assumes that firms can and should use external ideas as well as internal ideas to advance their technology" [13] embedded in the notion that the sources of knowledge for innovation is dispersed in the economy and involves a deliberately managed knowledge flows across organizational boundaries [62]. Through collaborative project partners develop, create and share knowledge. In dealing with different background, culture, process, and knowledge throughout collaborative project, organizations must improve their practices to access, share and create knowledge. Ecosystem of innovation [19, 20, 63] is more and more considered as territorial systems that facilitates and drive collaboration which facilitate knowledge sharing and innovation. Our results show that interprofessional collaboration- expressed by academia and industry partners- presents more challenge and obstacle in sharing knowledge. On the one hand lack of communication and leadership is often expressed as a missing skills of academia partners. On the other hand, a misunderstanding of the reality of partners is showed to be the reasons of those missing skills. This tensions between academia and industrials partners leads to a poor projects' output in terms of knowledge sharing whether is strong the contribution of governmental actors to bolster collaboration and open innovation.

5.3 A balanced bottom-up and top-down collaboration approach

Our results show the balance between a "top down" and a "bottom up" approach is required in order to promote collaboration between ecosystem actors. Despite the existence of social proximity and geographic proximity that should lead to facilitate knowledge sharing process, our informants expressed a weak knowledge sharing through those collaborative projects.

6. Conclusion

The purpose of this paper was to gain a better understanding of factors that impede and foster the inter-organizational knowledge sharing within a collaborative project. The results generated in this analysis highlight how social proximity, which is considerate as a facilitator to collaboration and interactive learning, is needed to initiate the collaborative project but neither fosters collaboration nor facilitates the knowledge sharing process in a lack of other factors. Contrary to research showing the relevant role of social proximity to foster collaboration, our finding suggests that within the project progress, the lack of leadership and interest in the project the collaborative project fail to achieve their goal which is the knowledge sharing. Furthermore, this paper contributes to existing literature on collaboration and knowledge management by analysing the role of proximity, especially social proximity, depending on project stage and progression. This paper points out the need of multilevel analysis to better understand the dynamic of interorganizational knowledge sharing. As stated earlier, three level of analysis used for this research. The three levels are continually interacting. Indeed, we believe that the relationships between organizations within the cluster impact the dynamics of individuals and groups that collaborate, but also these organizations evolve within an environment that shapes them. This impact is by no means a unilateral one, since the structures of social systems are both «conditions and results of the activities performed by agents who are part of these systems» ([64]: 15). There is therefore a duality between action and structure according to Giddens [64]. Similarly, as the knowledge sharing is a social phenomenon, we believe that the understanding of the interorganizational knowledge sharing dynamic within the cluster should shed light on the interaction between different actors and social systems at three level of the ecosystem: micro, meso and macro. The choice of CRIAQ projects as a single case of the study limits the generalization of the results. Moreover, even if the choice of this typical case seems adequate to our study and our research concerns, it would be interesting to study other cases of collaborative projects within the ecosystem. In addition, a comparison between national and international projects would make it possible to deepen certain results, in particular on the concepts of proximity, leadership and the philosophy of the organization.

Appendix 1: data structure

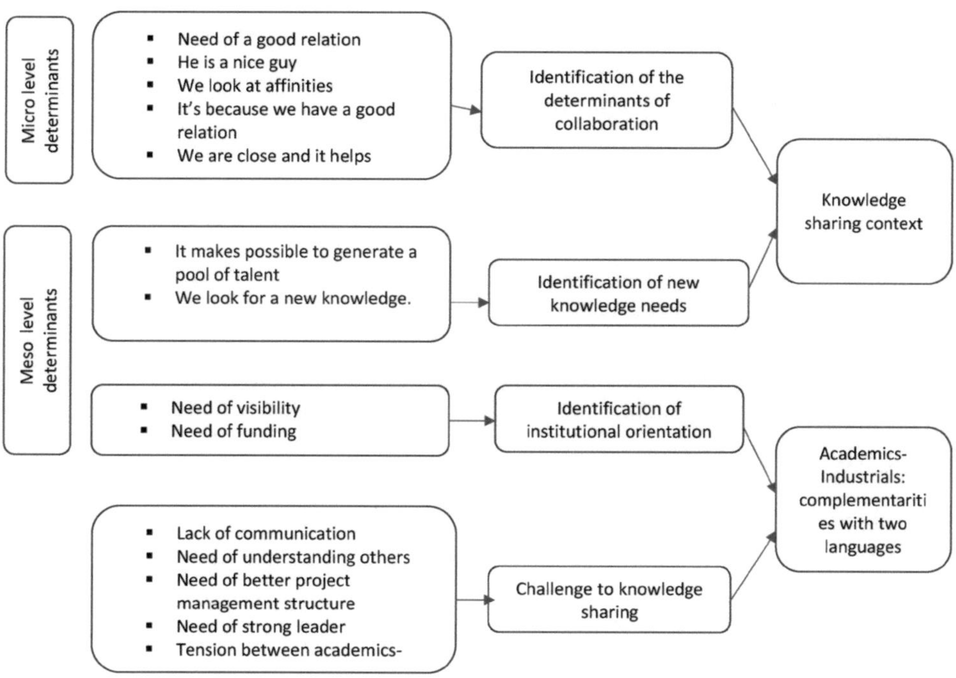

Author details

Chiraz Guedda
University of Montreal at Quebec, Montreal, Canada

*Address all correspondence to: guedda.chiraz@gmail.com

References

[1] Cohendet P, Parmentier G, Simon L: Managing knowledge, creativity and innovation» in *The Elgar Companion to Innovation and Knowledge Creation,* Elgar Editions; 2017; 197-214

[2] Harvey JF, Cohendet P, Simon L, Dubois LE: Another cog in the machine: Designing communities of practice in professional bureaucracies; *European Management Journal*, 2013; 31; 27-40

[3] Connel J, Kriz A, Thorpe, M: Industry clusters: an antidote for knowledge sharing and collaborative innovation?, *Journal of Knowledge Management*, 2014; Vol 18, Issue: 1; 137-151

[4] Feldman MP: The New Economics of Innovation, Spillovers and Agglomeration: A Review of Empirical Studies», *Economics of Innovation and New Technology*, 1999; Vol 8; 5-25.

[5] Lundvall BÅ: *National Systems of Innovation: Towards A Theory of Innovation and Interactive Learning,* Paperback Editions, 1995; 342p.

[6] Rallet A, Torre A: Geogrpahy of innovation, proximity and beyond, in *The Elgar Companion to Innovation and Knowledge Creation,* Elgar Editions,2017; 421-439

[7] Asheim BT, Boschma R, Cooke P: Constructing Regional Advantage: Platform Policies Based on Related Variety and Differentiated Knowledge Bases, *Regional Studies*, 2011; Vol 45; No.7; 893-904.

[8] Fritsch, M., et Slavtchev, V. 2011. «Determinants of the Efficiency of Regional Innovation Systems», *Regional Studies,* Vol. 45, No.7, p : 905-918.

[9] Huggins,R., Johnston, A., et Stride, C. 2012. « Knowledge networks and universities: Locational and organisational aspects of knowledge transfer interactions», *Entrepreneurship and Regional Development,* Vol.24, No:7-8, p : 475-502.

[10] Balland, PA, Boscham R, Frenken K: Proximities and Innovation: From Statics to Dynamics, *Regional Studies,* 2015; Vol 49

[11] Antonelli C: Collective Knowledge Communication and Innovation: The Evidence of Technological Districts, *Regional Studies*, 2000; Vol 34; No. 6; 535-547

[12] Hayek FA: The use of knowledge in society, *American Economic Review*, 1945; Vol 35; 519-530.

[13] Chesbrough H: *Open innovation*, Boston Editions, Mass.: Harvard Business School, 2003; 227 p.

[14] Hamel G, Doz Y, Prahalad CK: Collaborate with Your Competitors-and Win, *Harvard Business Review,* 1989; Vol 67, No. 1; 133-139

[15] Krugman P: *Geography and Trade*, Cambridge: MIT Press; 1991

[16] Porter M: Clusters and the new economics of Competition», *Harvard Business Review*, 1998; Vol 76, No 6, pp 77-90.

[17] Moore JF: The *Death of Competition: Leadership and Strategy in the Age of Business Ecosystems,* New York Editions: Harper Business, 1996; 279 p.

[18] Adner R, Kapoor, R: Value creation in innovation ecosystems: how the structure of technological interdependence affects firm performance in new technology generations. *Strategic Management Journal*, 2012; Vol. 3, 306-333.

[19] Adner R: Match Your Innovation Strategy to Your Innovation Ecosystem, *Havard Business Review*, 2006; 1-11

[20] Iansiti M, Levien R: *The Keystone Advantage: What the New Dynamics of Business Ecosystem Mean for Strategy, Innovation and Sustainability,* Harvard Business School Press, Boston, Massachusetts. 2004; 253p.

[21] Fujita M, Thisse J: *Economics of Agglomeration: Cities, Industrial Location, and Regional Growth*, Cambridge University Press, 2002

[22] OCDE: *Boosting Innovation: The Cluster Approach,* Édition: OECD Publishing, Paris; 1999

[23] Preissl B, Solimene L: *The Dynamics of Clusters and Innovation: beyond systems and networks*, Physica Verlag Editions, Heidelberg, New York,2003; 244 p.

[24] Becattini G: Le district marshallien: une notion socio-économique, in Benko et Lipietz: *Les régions qui gagnent*, Édition: Paris: PUF, 1992; 35-56.

[25] Brusco S: The Emilian model: productive decentralization and social integration, *Cambridge Journal of Economics*, 1982; Vol. 6, pp 167-184.

[26] Nonaka I: A dynamic theory of organizational knowledge creation, *Organization Science*, 1994; Vol 5, No.1, pp 14-37.

[27] Storper MS, Venables AJ: Buzz: face-to-face contact and the urban economy», *Journal of Economic Geography,* 2004; Vol 4; 51-370

[28] Cohendet P, Kirman AP, Zimmermann JB: Émergence, formation et dynamique des réseaux: modèles de la morphogenèse, *Revue d'Économie Industrielle*, 2003; No.103, 15-42.

[29] Nahapiet J, Gratton L, Rocha HO: Knowledge and relationships: when cooperation is the norm; *European Management Review*; 2005; Vol 2; 3-14.

[30] Brown J S, Duguid P: Organiztional learning and communities-of-practice: Toward a unified of working, learning and innovation, *Organization Science*, 1991; Vol2, No.1; 40-57.

[31] Uzzi B: Social structure and competition in interfirm networks: The paradox of embeddedness», *Administrative Science Quarterly*, 1997; Vol 42; 35-67.

[32] Granovetter MS: The strength of weak ties, *American Journal of Sociology*, 1973; Vol 78, No.6, 1360-1380.

[33] Boschma R A, Lambooy J G, Shutjens V: Embeddedness and innovation, in Taylor M. and LeonardS. (Eds) *Embedded Enterprise and Social Capital. International Perspectives*, 2002;19-35.

[34] Boschma, R A: Proximity and innovation: A critical assessment, *Regional Studies*, 2005; Vol 39; 61-74.

[35] Granovetter M: Economic action and social structure: The problem of embeddedness, *American Journal of Sociology*, 1985; Vol 91, No 3, pp 481-510.

[36] Asheim, B., Lars Coenen, L., et Moodysson, J. 2007. « Constructing knowledge-based regional advantage: implications for regional innovation policy», International Journal of Entrepreneurship and Innovation Management, Vol.7, No. 2-5, p : 140-155.

[37] Liu Y, Liang, L: Evaluating and developing resource-based operations strategy for competitive advantage: an exploratory study of Finnish high-tech manufacturing industries, International Journal of Production Research, 2015; 53:4, 1019-1037

[38] Corno F, Reinmoeller P, Nonaka I: Knowledge Creation within Industrial Systems», *Journal of Management and Governance,* Vol3, 1999; 379-394.

[39] Argote L, McEvily B, Reagans R: Managing Knowledge in Organizations:

An integrative Framework and Review of emerging Themes, 2003; *Management Science*, Vol 49, No.4, pp 571-582.

[40] Grant RM: 1996: Toward a knowledge-based theory of the firm, *Strategic Management Journal*, 1996; Vol 17, 109-122.

[41] Szulanski G: Exploring internal Stickiness: impediments to the transfer of the best practice within the firm, *Strategic Management Journal*, Vol. 17, winter special issue, 1996; 27-43.

[42] Reagans, R., McEvily, B. .2003. "Network structure and knowledge transfer: The effects of cohesion and range". Administrative Science Quarterly, Vol. 48(2), p240-267.

[43] Kogut B, Zander U: Knowledge of the firm and the evolutionary theory of the multinational corporation, *Journal of International Business Studies,* 1993; Vol 24, No. 4; 625-645.

[44] Nonaka I, Konno N: The concept of Ba: Building a foundation for Knowledge creation, *California Management Review*, 1998; Vol 40, No. 3; 40-54.

[45] Knight L: Network Learning: Exploring Learning by Interorganizational Networks; *Human Relations*, 2002; Vol 55, No.4; 427-454.

[46] Strauss AL: *La trame de la négociation: sociologie qualitative et interactionnisme*, Paris Editions L'Harmattan, 1992; 319 p.

[47] Wulf.A and Butel. L. 2017. Knowledge Sharing and Collaborative Relationships in Business Eco- systems and Networks: A Definition and a Demarcation. Industrial Management & Data Systems Vol. 117 (7), p: 1407-1425.

[48] Etzkowitz, H., et Leydesdorff, L. 2000. « The dynamics of innovation: from National Systems and "Mode 2" to a Triple Helix of university–industry–government relations», *Research policy,* Vol. 29, No.2, p:109-123.

[49] Yin, R. K. 2009. « *Case Study Research: Design and Methods»,* (4e ed), Los Angels : Sage Publications, 219 p.

[50] Eisenhardt KM: Building theory from case study research », *Academy of Management Review*, 1989; Vol 14, No.4; 532-550.

[51] Eisenhardt, KM, Graebner, ME: Theory Building from Cases: Opportunities and Challenges, *Academy of Management Review*, 2007; Vol 50, No:1, 25-32.

[52] Patton, M.Q. 2002. *«Qualitive Research and Evaluation Methods»,* Édition: Newbury Park; Sage Publications, 598p.

[53] Langley, A. 1999. «Strategies for Theorizing from Process Data», *Academy of Management Review,* Vol.24, No. 4, p : 691-710.

[54] Corbin J, Strauss, A: Grounded Theory Research: Procedures, Canons, and Evaluative Criteria, *Qualitative Sociology*, 1990; Vol 13, No.1; 3-21.

[55] Corley, KG, Gioia DA: Identity ambiguity and change in the wake of a corporate spin-off. *Administrative Science Quarterly*, 2004; Vol 49, No. 2; 173-208.

[56] Charmaz K: *Constructing Grounded Theory: A Practical Guide Through Qualitative Analysis*, Sage Publications; 2006.

[57] Miles, M.B., et Huberman.M. 2003. *« Analyse des données qualitatives ».* Édition De boeck, 626 p.

[58] Strauss, A., et Corbin, J. 2004. *« Les fondements de la recherche qualitative : techniques et procédures de développement de la théorie enracinée »,* Academic Press Fribourg, 342p

[59] Chesbrough. H. 2017. Foreword in Extreme Teaming: Lessons in Complex, Cross-Sector Leadership, By Amy C. Edmondson, Jean-François Harvey. Emerald Publishing, p: 9-12.

[60] Zhang Y, Chen K, Zhu G. et al: Inter-organizational scientific collaborations and policy effects: an ego-network evolutionary perspective of the Chinese Academy of Sciences; 2016; 1383-1415

[61] Edmondson AC, Harvey, JF: Extreme Teaming: Lessons in Complex, Cross-Sector Leadership. Bingley: Emerald Publishing Limited; 2017

[62] Chesbrough H, Bogers: Explicating Open Innovation: Clarifying an Emerging Paradigm for Understanding Innovation." In Henry Chesbrough, Wim Vanhaverbeke and Joel West, eds., *Open Innovation: New Frontiers and Application*s, Oxford: Oxford University Press; 2014

[63] Adner, R., et Kapoor, R. 2010. « Value creation in innovation ecosystems: how the structure of technological interdependence affects firm performance in new technology generations ». *Strategic Management Journal,* Vol. 3, p:306-333.

[64] Giddens A: *La constitution de la société: éléments de la théorie de la structuration*, PUF, 1987; 474p.

Chapter 12

Quality of Life in Employee with Workaholism

Ozlem Koseoglu Ornek and Nurcan Kolac

Abstract

Workaholism has been a growing issue among the labour force worldwide. However, there is no consensus between scholars about its definition yet. It might be described as "being overly concerned about work, driven by a strong and uncontrollable desire to work, and spending so much energy and effort on work that it impairs private relationships, personal hobbies/activities, and/or health". Generally, people with specific personality traits may have an increased chance of developing workaholism. In addition, there are other factors, such as sociocultural characteristics, relationships with colleagues and significant others, and organizational culture might also play an important influence on developing workaholism. It causes many physical and psychological health problems, such as high blood pressure, anxiety, depression, and family and lifestyle dissatisfaction, and a reduction in job satisfaction, presenteeism, and motivation. Putting all of this together, it is clear that workaholism has a negative influence on employees' quality of life and overall well-being. Therefore, this study aimed at examining a variety of approaches to define "workaholism" in related literature, defining its etiology, related factors, outcomes, prevention, and treatment. The PubMed/Medline database was also used for related studies that were published in English. "Workaholism", "obsessive–compulsive behavior", and "quality of health" were used as keywords. It is crucial to take action to prevent people from becoming workaholics. Early diagnoses of workaholism, using predictive factors by occupational healthcare professionals in the workplace, would help decrease its impact on workers' health, and an effective treatment of workaholism should be applied.

Keywords: workaholism, job productivity, obsessive–compulsive behavior, quality of health, and prevention

1. Introduction

The majority of the world's population works. Therefore, work plays an important role in their lives. For personal development and economic needs, it is the most important factor for people. However, working conditions and the way people approach their work life have a great impact on their quality of life and well-being. According to the literature review, workaholism is increasing rapidly compared to previous years, and thus, it seems that there is an increased interest in workaholism-related issues among researchers% [1–3]. In Norway, the recent study by Andreassen et al. [1] showed that the prevalence of workaholism was at 7.3%, but it may be that the rate of self-workaholism is much higher among the working population than it was estimated [2, 3]. Therefore, the amount of research associated with workaholism has been increasing in recent years, and the terms "work addiction", "workaholism", "excessively overwork" have been prevalent throughout [4–7]. However, it seems that there is no common consensus about its meaning, which may very well be considered an important public issue in the future; this is because it gradually deteriorates people's health, causing mental and physical health problems, such as coronary heart disease, anxiety, and work-related stress. For a long time now, it has also had a negative influence on people's social lives, including family relationships and work performance—resulting in the decreasing of quality of life and well-being. Workaholics tend to spend most of their time working, leaving aside their social life, which leads to having more family conflicts and a lack of recreational activities [3, 4]. These results can be explained by the fact that they constantly feel stressed and pressured to succeed, physically harming themselves due to their work hours. Beyond that, it has been stated that workaholics are more likely to have obsessive–compulsive disorder, attention-deficit disorder, and hyperactivity disorder, showing that workaholism may be a sign of deeper psychological or emotional problems.

Although much is known about the consequences of workaholism, there is very little information about the source of workaholism [3–5].

Therefore, this review was aimed to examine definitions of "workaholism", the factors affecting the occurrence of workaholism, and the consequences of workaholism.

2. Method

It was aimed to examine a variety of approaches to define workaholism in related literature; it also seeks to define, and discuss its etiology, related factors, outcomes, prevention, and its treatment subsequently. The PubMed/Medline database was used for reviewing related studies published in English. "Workaholism", "obsessive–compulsive behavior", and "quality of health" were used as keywords. There were no restrictions in place regarding setting, study design, or timeline.

3. Workaholism

The term "workaholism" originally derived from the word "alcoholism". It is seen as type of addiction, similar to gambling and sex. According to written literature, it was first coined and used in 1971 by Wayne E. Oates. It was initially described as "addiction to work, the compulsive and uncontrollable need to work incessantly", asserting that workaholism is an addiction to work and has many common connections to alcoholism. At this time, workaholism was simply defined by Oates [3] as "*a person whose need for work has become so excessive that it creates noticeable disturbance or interference with his bodily health, personal happiness, and interpersonal relationships, and with his smooth social functioning*" [3]. However, compared to other common addictions, such as gambling or drug use, the definition of work addiction is still being developed through a variety of discussion, thought, or confusion [4–6]. In last half century, workaholism, as a term, has been widely used in related literature. For example, it was defined workaholism according to working hours per week. Nevertheless, this approach can easily meet resistance, particularly in developing and undeveloped countries where people commonly work more than what the definition states. At this point, some writers argue that simply focusing on the criteria of time is not enough to define people as "workaholics" [8]. Machlowitz defined "workaholism" as an approach or attitude toward working instead of explaining it with just the amount of time put in at work, since it is well known that "workaholics" keep thinking about work even when they are not there. A qualitative study was conducted with more than 100 workaholics, and the results showed that these workers were happy and satisfied with their life [9]. However, as it has been stated, there are a variety of different approaches for defining "workaholism", with no consensus regarding the term. Some scientists present workaholism in positive terms and images by stressing the benefits from a high work investment, including extra work effort [9, 10], but others present it in negative terms and have emphasized the riskier sides, including health and "work-life conflicts" [3–7, 10, 11]. The writers who view workaholism negatively term interpreted "workaholism" as being equal to other addictions. Thus, they have focused on its detrimental effects. For example, Cherrington views workaholism as a preposterous dedication to extreme work [12]. On the other hand, some writers see "workaholism" as a decisive individual characteristic [13–15]. It is also possible, through the literature [16], to define "workaholism" using four distinguished aspects:

- Robinson and Scott define workaholism behaviourally [13, 17], and Machlowitz, Spence, and Robinson define it attitudinally [9, 14].

- Killinger, Oates, and Robinson view workaholism as an addiction [3, 18, 19].

- It is considered positive [9, 10] or negative [3, 17, 20].

- It is acknowledged as having different types with various antecedents and outcomes [13, 14, 21, 22].

Spence and Robinson [14] define "workaholism" as a set of varied attitudes and behavioral patterns. The patterns consist of high levels of psychological involvement with work, intrinsic drive to work, and low or no work enjoyment (a high level of enjoyment describes an enthusiastic workaholic, and a low level of enjoyment describes a workaholic) [14]. According to them, the workaholic who is "highly work involved, feels compelled or driven to work because of inner pressures and is low in enjoyment of work". Their definition of workaholism has been widely used and accepted in the literature. They have used "workaholic triad" as a measurement of workaholism. The triad consists of three dimensions: "work involvement", "feeling driven to work", and "work enjoyment". They identify three types of workaholics based on the scores from the dimensions. The workaholic dimension types are "work addict", "work enthusiast", and "enthusiastic work addict". For instance, the person in the "work enjoyment" category has a low work addiction score, but the "work involvement" and "feeling driven to work" dimensions have a high work addiction score. "Work enthusiasts" get a high work addiction score from the "work involvement" and "work enjoyment" dimensions, but they receive a low work addiction score from the "feeling driven to work" dimension [14]. However, "enthusiastic work addicts" get a high work addiction score from all three dimensions. They have also defined six sub-types of workaholics and non-workaholics, which are "work addicts", "enthusiastic workaholics", "work enthusiast", "disenchanted workers", "relaxed workers", and "unengaged workers". Each of them shows a different level of reaction based on the dimensions mentioned above [22] (see **Table 1**). Compared to other sub-types of the workaholics, "work addicts" are expected to be perfectionists, to experience higher levels of stress, and to complain more about physical health problems. Machlowitz has brought similar themes with her. She alleged that "what set workaholics apart is their attitude towards work, not

Workaholics' sub-types	Dimension of workaholism		
	Feeling driven to work	Work enjoyment	Work involvement
Workaholic	High	Low	High
Enthusiastic workaholic	High	High	High
Work enthusiast	Low	High	High
Relaxed worker	Low	High	Low
Disgruntled worker	High	Low	Low
Uninvolved worker	Low	Low	Low

Table 1.
Dimension of workaholism and workaholics' sub-types.

the number of hours they work". According to her, the definition relies on "physic income", which is based on responsibility, sense, opportunity, and recognition (not monetary) [9]. Later, Buelens and Poelmans reiterate Spence and Robinson's six-sub types of workaholics and developed it further, identifying the "reluctant hard worker" as an additional sub-type, while also speculating that "alienated professionals" might be an additional sub-type [21].

"Workaholism" is also defined as a person who spends an excessive amount time at work, resulting in a deterioration of family, social relationships, and recreational needs. It is argued that a workaholic has some specific characteristics, such as spending substantial unprompted time in work activities, thinking about the job when not at work, and working beyond organizational or economical requirements [14]. In their defense of the concept "Work beyond organizational or economical requirements", they think that the organizational work pressure leads people to work more, but if this effort is beyond what is logically expected it should be considered workaholism. So, in the workaholic organization people are expected to "work hard", but if the work expectation—based on the organization's criteria—is not met, workers do not have many choices except leaving work or being dismissed. Thus, the result of the organizational requirement can vary. It depends on the workers, but if the workers have no choice other than accepting to meet the standards of the workaholic organization, they will be appropriately considered to be a workaholic. They stated that the workaholic may indicate one of the workaholism patterns, which have been classified by them [14]:

- *Compulsive-dependent workaholic*: It is claimed that people who are compulsive-dependent workaholics will most likely have positive associations with the level of stress, anxiety, physical and psychological well-being, and health, but they will also have negative associations with job performance and job-life satisfaction. It can be interpreted that the more the worker is a compulsive-dependent workaholic the more the worker tends to have a poor quality of life.

- *Perfectionist workaholic:* Generally, people who have an obsessive–compulsive disorder exhibit a perfectionist personality. So, perfectionists may be very likely to have problems in their relationships at work, with their families, and in their social lives. They hold a very high standards for themselves and for their goals; they are also success-oriented at work, and their levels of stress and anxiety are high. Shortly, perfectionists may have a low quality of life and well-being in long time. According to Scott et al., a "perfectionist workaholic" will correlate positively with the levels of physical and psychological health, stress, antagonistic interpersonal relationships, voluntary turnover and absenteeism, and low job performance and satisfaction. Naughton presents a focused approach with this pattern. He explains that "workaholism" is based on two dimensions: "obsession compulsion" and "career commitment" [23].

- *Achieve-oriented workaholic:* It is a very likely possible to see obsessive–compulsive disorder in one's health records. These workers relate positively to health problems, job and life satisfaction, job performance, low voluntary turnover, and pro-social behavior.

They claim that long working hours do not necessarily characterize workaholics. Douglas and Morris claim that "working long hours is a behavioural pattern, which is likely triggered by certain attitudes". Additionally, there might be a variety of reasons for working long hours and maybe only some of them would be considered workaholism; for example, people who have a high work involvement and attitude are predisposed to work long hours and are, therefore, more inclined to suffer from workaholism [16].

Snir and Zohar define "workaholism" as an individual's consistent and considerable designation of time to work-related activities and thoughts that are not derived from external necessities. According to them, there are some advantages to this definition over the others. For example, this definition is consistency, which means that workaholism should result from a temporary, heavy workload. Additionally, it also considers external necessities (e.g., working overtime to pay off debt or working long hours to advance one's career), and focuses on values and attitudes [8]. It is based on the core elements of workaholism, discussed above. At this point, it is likely to see a common approach in some of the other writers' definition of workaholism. For instance, they suggested that workaholics have three main characteristics: addiction, obsession, and driven to work due to internal needs, not external [3, 11, 18, 24]. Hakanen and Peters suggested a different approach to defining workaholism, comparing the typology of workaholics and engaged workers. They argued that workaholics are much more prone to invest their resources—such as attention, emotions, time, and energy—in work even if it hurts their social and private life. The workaholics will continue this behavioral pattern regardless of whether they fail or succeed. The workaholics' behavior and mindset are on focused on work even when they are not at work [25]. When the "workaholism" definition is critiqued, described by variety of writers since 1971, "long working hours" is still a controversial component. In recent studies, the component has been discussed in detail. For example, the definition by Griffiths and Ng, along with the definition by Sorensen and Feldman, have developed a more contemporary definition, including a steady pattern of "high work investment", "long working hours", and working obsessively without organizational requirements [6, 26].

In the academic literature, the concept of long working hours generally reminds others of Japan, because the reason for working "long working hours" is simply the demand of employers or the desire of the workers—it is a part of a socio-cultural issue. For the Japanese, it is about fulfilling their duties to society, which they think they owe to themselves and their social being [27]. Recently, Robinson defined four types of workaholism: *The blumic:* "who makes it a point to do the job perfectly or not at all"; *the relentless:* "who are compulsively driven to work quickly and meet deadlines, and who find it difficult to stop working"; *the savoring:* "who are consumed by a preoccupation with details"; and *the attention-deficit:* "who start numerous projects/ventures but become easily dulled and restless, continually motivated to seek further challenges" [7]. In one of the recent definitions of workaholism, Wojdylo described it as a pathological work style and addiction disorder. Wojdylo has used the term *"work craving" when defining workaholism. According to her, workaholism is comprised of a "obsessive–compulsive component", "anticipation of self-worth compensatory incentives from work", "anticipation of relief from negative affect or withdrawal symptoms resulting from working", and "neurotic perfectionism"* [28]. As it can be seen, "workaholism" typologies have been rarely discussed, based on theory or empirical studies.

3.1 Workaholism etiology/factors related with workaholism

There are a variety of factors that presumably induce and maintain workaholism. Some central theories and factors that may result in driven people falling into workaholism will be explained subsequently in the next paragraphs.

Workaholism may be associated with internal fundamental psychological needs for self-autonomy and competence. It is known that these fundamental internal needs have influence on developing people's behavior [29]. Thus, workaholism might be correlated with these needs. For instance, when a person feels incompetent, that person will try hard to feel competent, which could be work-related, too. So, this obsession with work may be related to one's unsatisfied needs. On the other hand, there are studies indicating that workaholism is also related to external behavior, such as the avoidance of criticism from people around them [30]. In this case, people hold high standards and ambitious work objectives, always trying to complete the best of their work, while avoiding their managers or co-workers to avoid any criticism. This approach and behavior may also relate to an obsessive–compulsive personality. Beyond that, it seems that there is a strong relationship between the personality and workaholism. Pitrowski and Vadanovich put forth that workaholism is developed from the integration of individual factors, such as personality traits and home and family characteristics; this includes roles, responsibilities, demanding internal and external factors (such as the appreciation of earning more money, either at home or at work, at first) [31]. Some studies explain the etiology of workaholism with personality traits such as "neuroticism", "conscientiousness", "narcissism", and "perfectionism" [32–35]. Furthermore, "obsessive-compulsion", "achievement orientation", "perfectionism", and "conscientiousness" personality traits have a strong link to workaholism. "Perfectionism", "preoccupation with orderliness", "mental and interpersonal control", "openness", and "efficiency" are main characteristics of an obsessive–compulsive personality disorder [36]. A study concluded that "rigid perfectionism" is a core component of an obsessive–compulsive personality [37]. People who have an obsessive–compulsive personality chronically experience a variety of difficulties in their social and work lives. This type of personality may help lead people to becoming workaholics. In line with this, one study found that there were two aspects of an obsessive–compulsive personality that were prevalent in workaholism: feeling elevated levels of responsibility and being quietly stubborn [38]. Also, learned family values and intrinsic work values may relate to workaholism [26, 39]. Socio-cultural experiences, such as a stressful childhood and behavioral reinforcements that include tangible or intangible rewards, experiences of a "winner-takes-all system", and an organizational environment can be precursor to workaholism [26]. "Joy in working", "guilt and anxiety when not working", "obsession with working", and "working long hours" are defined as the immediate precursors to workaholism [40]. Additionally, some sociodemographic characteristics may lead to developing workaholism. For example, workaholism was found to be less likely among young blue-collar workers [41]; however, a study showed that there were no meaningful differences of workaholism found among gender, race, or age [42]. Beyond that, Beiler-May suggested that women, in reality, are more prone to workaholism than men [43]. Similar gender differences were found by other studies [14, 44]. Compared to men, women suffer from societal norms and restrictions, along with a higher responsibility for the (extra workload) [45]. Particularly, married women workers tend to have a second round of work at home by taking responsibility for the family and children. These barriers may prevent women from spending more time at work, therefore developing workaholism, as well [46, 47]. Nevertheless, it is claimed in other studies that men work relatively longer hours, which may cause them to be a workaholic [48].

Cognitive perspectives, psychological addiction models, and social and learning theories have also been used for explaining workaholism. According to the cognitive perspective, "basic cognitions", such as supposition, expectancies, attributions, and automatic thoughts, are presumed to activate workaholic behavior [49]. Therefore, if a worker has a low-self-image and has a belief that working hard makes a person successful, the worker may then show workaholic behavior. Positive self-efficacy [50] might also be tied to the explanation of workaholism. If a worker thinks that he/she has a better positive efficacy at work more than outside (home or social life), he/she may prioritize work. Some studies tested cognitive perspective. For example, high self-efficacy was correlated with workaholism [44], driven in work was negatively regarded with self-esteem [49], and passive avoidance and depressive reactions were associated with an obsessive work drive [32]. In a study with administrative staff from a university, a cross-sectional structural model was examined. It concluded that enthusiastic workaholics high in self-efficacy showed high autonomy, mental competence, and emotional competence, but in turn it leads to subsequent workaholism [51].

Many scholars from the field of addiction obviously claim that workaholism is an addiction [16, 40, 52]. The medical addiction model explains the physical dependence on a substance. When the substance is absent, dependent people crave the substance and may show symptoms of withdrawal syndrome [43]. Thus, scholars from the addiction field claim that the concept of workaholism works with the concept of addiction [32].

The learning theory explains workaholism using normal learning principles [53]. According to the theory, if the conditions of workaholism are present, it can cause anyone to become a workaholic. The behavior of workaholics appears and is reinforced if the similar behaviors result in positive outcomes, such as praise from supervisors and a salary increase, or if it has led to negative outcomes, such as conflicts at home and bored with leisure time [7]. The social learning theory explains workaholic behavior: if a worker observes and sees the benefits in the behaviors of significant others (e.g., family members, managers, and leaders) leading to positive results, a workaholic's behavior can be affected, mirroring them to reach desired outcomes.

Additionally, some researchers think that family perspective [54] and behavioral reinforcement, from an aetiological perspective [55], are prominent in developing workaholism. For example, family is central in an individual's life, where one's personality is built up and progressed. There are times when working long hours may equal that of caring for their family, which is seen as high in responsibility. Thus, this can possibly develop into workaholism. For example, in a student-led study, it was concluded that students who had a high workaholism score described their parents as hard-workers, and vice-versa for those who had a low workaholism score. On the other hand, behavioral reinforcements, such as organizational reward systems, satisfaction, complaints, and compliments, may lead to workaholism [24, 26, 55].

3.2 Workaholism outcomes

Workaholism has a variety of negative consequences. These are briefly related to work life, social and family life, and physical and psychological health. In the long-term, the influence of workaholism can negatively impact quality of life and well-being. In the following paragraphs, the overview of workaholism's consequences will be discussed with reference to empirical studies.

Workaholics tend to have family problems. For example, workaholics experience a relatively high amount of work–family conflict [56–58], greater marital estrangement [59], feelings of being unsuccessful, being ineffective in solving family problems [2], rigid relationships with children and/or spouse [60], and children of workaholic parents have a higher level of psychological health problems, such as depression and external locus of control, compared to non-workaholic parents. It was reported that compared to men, female workaholics are relatively unlikely to get married [61].

Studies show that the negative life outcomes due to workaholism can be seen in all parts of life. These negative outcomes are perceived high stress [63–66], low self-esteem, low self-efficacy, low life-satisfaction, sleeping problems (e.g., insomnia or weak sleep) [63, 67–69], psychological distress [28], career dissatisfaction, poor job performance [70, 71], burnout [25, 72, 73], and higher amount of work–family conflict [74]. Additionally, a study conducted in Spain has supported the negative consequences discussed above. The study concluded that personality traits such as engagement, obsessive–compulsiveness, and life and life-style dissatisfaction were strong predictive factors of workaholism [75]. Furthermore, other negative consequences of workaholism include poor or worsening social functions [76], taking sick-leave [77], high blood pressure, cardiovascular risk [21, 78], obsessive–compulsive disorder, anxiety, depression [21, 79, 80], and physical pain [76, 80–82].

As a result, it appears that an internal obsessive work drive is a core element of workaholism correlated with many negative consequences. In addition, it has been found that workaholism is related to a decreasing psychological well-being, happiness in life, perceptions of health and happiness [51, 81], and self-reported work performance [81].

3.3 Prevention and treatment of workaholism

It seems that the occurrence of workaholism will be an increasing trend. Thus, first, it is crucial to take action to prevent workaholism. Second, effective treatment of workaholism should be applied, but related literature tends to be insufficient due to the lack of randomized and experiment-control designed studies. However, there are some prevention and treatment approaches that have been promoted in the related literature. In the following paragraphs, the approaches are given.

Prevention of workaholism among workers is an important issue. Regarding workaholism and its consequences, it could begin with increasing the awareness of academics, employers, workers, members of occupational health, and all other members of the community. Then, screening programs should be regularly applied at the workplace for diagnosing potential workaholics. Workaholics or potential workaholics should be under treatment and followed-up on regularly. Indeed, factors that are predisposed to workaholism should be found and adjusted as much as possible, especially since some factors are possibly not easily adjusted. Nevertheless, Sussman provides a systematic approach in the prevention of workaholism. He suggested that prevention of workaholism should comprise all extents of life, including levels of society, organization or organizational roles, and individual characteristics. Possible examples of effective prevention at the society level include providing the possibility of protecting and highlighting the importance of "work-family-personal life" balance, making employers close the workplace during national holidays in order to promote the need for recreation and personal interests, while using public service advertisements and virtual campaigns that combat workaholism.

From the organizational level, an "Employee Assistance Program" can be used in the workplace. Workers should be encouraged to use vacation time, providing an opportunity for better engagement with the workplace and flexible roles in life [73, 83]. Periodic assessment can be applied at the workplace for examining workers' happiness, job satisfaction, and needs, which can be used for addressing situations before they get worse. From the view of the individual, features that are predisposed to workaholism should be addressed and effective correction programs should be applied. For instance, one useful approach may be for employers to promote opportunities for recreation that restrict "work-family-personal" life overlap. Another important argument for preventing workaholism is the effects on children of workaholic parents. These children should be taught how to watch themselves for any indications of developing "workaholism"—being involved in group discussions might be helpful.

There are several treatment approaches that have been discussed in the related literature, summarized in a study by Andreassen [7]. Firstly, a clinical assessment should be completed for treating workaholism. After that, among treatment approaches used for workaholism, "Cognitive Behavioral Therapy" is well-documented and found to be effective for behavioral addictions [84]. It helps workaholics by setting limits; for instance, time-management principles can be used. A second treatment method is "Motivational Interviewing" [85]. The "Motivational Interviewing" program consists of ground principles— *"show empathy, develop discrepancy, role with resistance, avoid argumentation and confrontation, support efficacy" —and* communication skills— *"open questions, affirmations, reflections and summations"*, and strategies [7]. Another treatment method is "Positive psychology" [86]. This method focuses on strengths and positive human qualities rather than on inadequacy and negativity. The fourth and last treatment method is "Anonymous Workaholic". It consists of a 12-step program. This method can be found worldwide on the internet, and people can benefit by attending online and offline meetings [87].

4. Conclusion

An overview of workaholism has been provided in this section. Despite a high prevalence of workaholism among the working population, not much is known about the issue. There is still not a consensus on its definition from the basis of science. The reasons people are driven into workaholism are relatively numerous and quite complex, including obsessive-compulsiveness, perfectionism, narcissism, sociocultural environment, and family and organizational characteristics (and so on). It appears that there is a great need for longitudinal and randomized control design studies for observing and examining the behaviors and health of workaholics.

Conflict of interest

There are no known direct or indirect potential competing interests relating to this work from any of the listed authors.

Financial support

The study was not supported or funded by any company.

Author details

Ozlem Koseoglu Ornek[1*] and Nurcan Kolac[2]

1 Occupational and Environmental Epidemiology and Net Teaching Unit, Institute and Outpatient Clinic for Occupational, Social and Environmental Medicine, Hospital of the Ludwig-Maximilian-University (LMU), Munich, Germany

2 Nursing Department, Faculty of Health Sciences, Marmara University, Istanbul, Turkey

*Address all correspondence to: ozlem.koseoglu62@gmail.com; ozlem.koseoglu@med.uni-muenchen.de

References

[1] Andreassen CS, Nielsen MB, Gjerstad J. International Journal of Stress Management and Workaholism : Findings From a Nationally. Int J Stress Manag [Internet]. 2017;Advance on. Available from: http://dx.doi.org/10.1037/str0000073

[2] Matuska KM. Workaholism, life balance, and well-being: a comparative analysis. J Occup Sci. 2010;17(2):104-11

[3] Oates WE. Confessions of a workaholic: The facts about work addiction. Cleveland: World Publishing Company; 1971

[4] Burke RJ. Workaholic Behaviors : Do Colleagues Agree ? Int J Stress Manag. 2007;14(3):312-20

[5] Atroszko PA,Demetrovics Z .Beyond the myths about wowr addiction : Toward a consensus on definition and trajectories for future studies on problematic overworking . A response to the commentories on: Ten myths about work addiction(Griffiths et al.,2018).Journal of Behavioral Addictions.2019; 8(1):7-15 https:// doi.org/10.1556/2006.8.2019.11

[6] Sussman S, Lisha N, Griffiths M. Prevalence of the addictions: A problem of the majority or the minority? Eval Health Prof. 2011;34:3-56

[7] Andreassen CS. Workaholism : An overview and current status of the research. J Behav Addict. 2014;3(5015):1-11

[8] Snir R, Harpaz I. The workaholism phenomenon: a cross-national perspective. Career Dev Int. 2006;11(5):369-73

[9] Machlowitz M. Workaholics: Living With Them, Working With Them. MA: Addison-Wesley, Reading; 1980

[10] Cantarow E. "Women workaholics." Mother Jones. 1979;6:56

[11] Porter G. Organizational impact of workaholism: Suggestions for researching the negative outcomes of excessive work. ournal Occup Heal Psychol. 1996;1(1):70-84

[12] Cherrington DJ. The work ethic: Working values and values that work. Amacom; 1980

[13] Scottl KS, Moore KS, Miceli MP. An exploration of the meaning and consequences of workaholism. Hum relations. 1997;50(3):287-314

[14] Spence JT, Robbins AS. Workaholism: definition, measurement, and preliminary results. J Pers Assess. 1992;58(1):160-78

[15] Malinowska, D., Tokarz, A. Workaholism Components in Relation to Life and Work Values. Int J Ment HealthAddiction 2019. https://doi.org/10.1007/s11469-019-00089-y

[16] Douglas EJ, Morris RJ. Workaholic, or just hard worker? Career Dev Int. 2006;11(5):394-417

[17] Robinson BE. Workaholism: Bridging the gap between workplace, sociocultural, and family research. J Employ Couns. 2000;37(1):31-47

[18] Killinger B. Workaholics: The Respectable Addicts. New York:NY: Killinger, Barbara; 1991

[19] Robinson BE. Typology of Workaholics with Implications for Counselors. J Addict Offender Couns. 2000;21(1):34-48

[20] Seybold, Karen Colapietro and PRS. Understanding Workaholism: A Review of Causes and Counselling Approaches. J Couns Dev. 1994;73(1):4-9

[21] Buelens M, Poelmans SA. Enriching the Spence and Robbins' Typology of Workaholism: Demographic, Motivational and Organizational Correlates. J Organ Chang Manag. 2004;17(5):440-58

[22] McMillan LH, O'driscoll MP, Marsh N V., Brady EC. Understanding Workaholism: Data Synthesis, Theoretical Critique and Future Design Strategies. Int J Stress Manag. 2001;8(2):69-91

[23] Naughton TJ. A Conceptual View of Workaholism and Implications for Career Counseling and Research. Career Dev Q. 1987;35(3):180-7

[24] Fassel D. Working Ourselves to Death: The High Costs of Workaholism, The Rewards of Recovery. Francisco: Harper San; 1990

[25] Hakanen JJ, Peeters MCW, Schaufeli WB. Different Types of Employee Well-Being Across Time and Their Relationships With Job Crafting. J Occup Health Psychol. 2018;23(2):289-301

[26] Ng TW, Sorensen KL, Feldman DC. Dimensions, antecedents, and consequences of workaholism: A conceptual integration and extension. ournal Organ Behav Int J Ind Occup Organ Psychol Behav. 2007;28(1):111-36

[27] Snir R, Harpaz I, Burke R. Workaholism in oraganizations: new research directions. Career Dev Int. 2006;11(5):369-74

[28] Wojdylo K, Karlsson W, Baumann N. Do I feel ill because I crave for work or do I crave for work because I feel ill ? A longitudinal analysis of work craving , self-regulation , and health. J Behav Addict. 2016;5(1):90-9

[29] Deci EL, Ryan RM. The "what" and "why" of goal pursuits: Human needs and the self determination of behavior. Psychol Inq. 2000;11(4):227-68

[30] Klink JJL Van Der, Blonk RWB, Schene AH, Dijk FJH Van. The Benefits of Interventions for Work-Related Stress. Am J Public Health. 2001;91(2)

[31] Piotrowski C, Vodanovich SJ. The interface between workaholism and work-family conflict: A review and conceptual framework. Organ Dev J. 2006;24(4):84-92

[32] Andreassen CS, Hetland JØRN, Pallesen STÅLE. Coping and workaholism. Results from a large cross-occupational sample. Testing, Psychom Methodol Appl Psychol. 2012;19:1-10

[33] Falco A, Girardi D,Di Sipio, A, Calvo V, Marogna C, Snir R. Is narcissism associated with heavy work investment? The moderating role of workload in the relationship between narcissism, workaholism, and work engagement. Int. J. Environ. Res. Public Health. 2020; 17:4750

[34] Avanzi L, Perinelli E, Vignoli M, Junker NM, Balducci C. Unravelling Work Drive: A Comparison between Workaholism and Overcommitment. İnternational Journal of Environmental Research and Public Health. [Internet] 2020; 17,5755 :2-14. Available from Doi: 10.3390/ijerph17165755

[35] Andreassen C, Schou JH, Pallesen S. The relationship between workaholism, basic needs satisfaction at work and personality. Eur J Pers. 2010;24:3-17

[36] American Psychiatric Association. Diagnostic and Statistical Manual for Mental Disorders. 5th ed. Washington, DC: American Psychiatric Association; 2013

[37] Liggett J, Sellbom M. Examining the DSM-5 Alternative Model of Personality Disorders Operationalization of

Obsessive – Compulsive Personality Disorder in a Mental Health Sample. Personal Disord Theory, Res Treat. 2018;9(5):397-407

[38] Mudrack PE. Job involvement, obsessive-compulsive personality traits, and workaholic behavioral tendencies. J Organ Chang Manag. 2004;17(5):490-508

[39] Liang Y-W, Chu C-M. Personality traits and personal and organizational inducements: Antecedents of workaholism. Soc Behav Personal an Int J. 2009;37(5):645-60

[40] Sussman S. Workaholism: A Review. J Addict Res Ther. 2013;6(1):1-18

[41] Kanai A, Wakabayashi M. Workaholism among Japanese blue-collar employees. Int J Stress Manag. 2001;8(2):129-45

[42] Porter G. Workaholic tendencies and the high potential for stress among co-workers. Int J Stress Manag. 2001;8(2):147-64

[43] Brown RIF. Some contributions of the study of gambling to the study of other addictions. Gambl Behav Probl Gambl. 1993;241-72

[44] Burke RJ, Matthiesen SB, Pallesen S. Workaholism, organizational life and well-being of Norwegian nursing staff. Career Dev Int [Internet]. 2006;11(5):463-77. Available from: http://dx.doi.org/10.1108/1362043061068305234

[45] Beiler-may A, Williamson RL, Clark MA, Carter NT. Gender Bias in the Measurement of Workaholism. J Pers Assess. 2017;99(1):104-10

[46] Wharton AS, Blair-Loy M. 'overtime culture' in a global corporation: a cross-national study of finance professionals' interest in working part-time. Work Occup. 2002;29(1):32-63

[47] Pirtman JF, Orthner DK. Gender differences in the prediction of job commitment. J Soc Behav Pers. 1988;3(4):227-48

[48] Harpaz I, Snir R. Workaholism: Its definition and nature. Hum relations. 2003;56(3):291-319

[49] Beck JS. Cognitive therapy. Basics and beyond. Guilford press; 2011

[50] Bandura A. Social cognitive theory of moral thought and action. Handb moral Behav Dev Psychol Press. 2014;69-128

[51] Líbano M del, Llorens S, Salanova M, Schaufeli W. Validity of a brief workaholism scale. Psicothema. 2010;22(1):143-50

[52] Goodman A. Addiction: Definitions and implications. Br J Addict. 1990;85(11):1403-8

[53] Skinner BF. About behaviorism. Vintage; 2011

[54] Robinson BE. Chained to the desk: A guidebook for workaholics, their partners and children, and the clinicians who treat them. NYU Press; 2014

[55] Van Wijhe C, Peeters M, Schaufeli W, Hout M van den. Understanding workaholism and work engagement: The role of mood and stop rules. Career Dev Int. 2011;16(3):254-70

[56] Huyghebaert T, Conseil AD, Beltou N, Gimenes G, Gillet N. Examining the Longitudinal Effects of Workload on Ill-Being Through Each Dimension of Workaholism. Int J Stress Manag [Internet]. 2018;25(2):144-62. Available from: http://dx.doi.org/10.1037/str0000055

[57] Andreassen CS, Griffiths MD, Gjertsen SR, Krossbakken E, Kvam S, Pallesen S. The relationships between

behavioral addictions and the five-factor model of personality. J Behav Addict. 2013;2(2):90-9

[58] Russo JA, Waters LE. Workaholic worker type differences in work in family conflict. Career Dev Int [Internet]. 2006;11(5):418-39. Available from: http://dx.doi.org/10.1108/13620430610683052

[59] Robinson BE, Carroll JJ, Flowers C. Marital estrangement, positive affect, and locus of control among spouses of workaholics and spoused of nonworkaholics:A national study. Am J Fam Ther. 2001;29(5):397-410

[60] Robinson BE. Work addiction: Implications for EAP counseling and research. Empl Assist Q. 1997;12(4):1-13

[61] Robinson BE, Kelley L. Adult children of workaholics: Self-concept, anxiety, depression, and locus of control. Am J Fam Ther. 1998;26(3):223-38

[62] Andreassen CS, Ursin H, Eriksen HR. The relationship between strong motivation to work, "workaholism", and health. Psychol Heal. 2007;22(5):615-29

[63] Yang X,Qiu D, Lau Mason CM, Lau TF.J The mediation role of work-life balance stress and chronic fatigue in the relationship between workaholism and depression among Chinese male workers in Hong Kong. Journal of Behavioral Addictions. 2020; 483-490 https://doi.org/10.1556/2006.2020.0002

[64] Andreassen CS, Hetland J, Molde H, Pallesen S. Workaholism and potential outcomes inwell-being and health in a cross-occupational sample. Stress Heal. 2011;27(3):209-14

[65] Psenicy A, Perat M. Fear of relation loss: Attachment Style as a vulnerability factor in job burnout. Sloven Journal of Public Health 2020; 59(3). Available from Doi: https:// doi.org/10.2478/sjph2020-0019

[66] Kovalchuk LS, Buono C, Emanuela Ingusci E, Maiorano F, De Carlo E, Andreina Madaro A Spagnoli P. Can Work Engagement be a resource for reducing workaholism's undesirable outcomes? A multiple mediating model ıncluding moderated mediation analysis. İnt.J Environ. Res. Public Health .2019;16(1402):2-20

[67] Burke RJ. Workaholism, self-esteem, and motives for money. Psychol Rep. 2004;94(2):457-63

[68] Burke RJ, Oberklaid F, Burgess Z. Workaholism among Australian women psychologists: antecedents and consequences. Women Manag Rev. 2004;19(5):252-9

[69] Mazzeti G, Schaufeli WB, Guglielmi D. Are Workaholics Born or Made ? Relations of Workaholism With Person Characteristics and. Int J Stress Manag. 2014;21(3):227-54

[70] Graves LM, Ruderman MN, Ohlot PJ, Weber TJ. Driven to work and enjoyment of work: Effects on managers' outcomes. J Manage. 2012;38(5):1655-80

[71] Holland DE, Vanderboom CE, Delgado AM, Weiss ME, Monsen KA. Describing pediatric hospital discharge planning care processes using the Omaha System. Appl Nurs Res [Internet]. 2016;30:24-8. Available from: http://dx.doi.org/10.1016/j.apnr.2015.08.009

[72] Schaufeli WB, Taris TW, Rhenen W Van. Workaholism, burnout, and work engagement: Three of a kind or three different kinds of employee well-being? Appl Psychol. 2008;57(2):173-203

[73] Brauchli R, Bauer GF, Hämmig O. Relationship between

time-based work-life conflict and burnout. Swiss J Psychol. 2011;70:165-73. Management Journal 2019;3:413-432 https//doi.org/10.1111/17488583.12235.

[74] Aziz S, Zickar MJ. A Cluster Analysis Investigation of Workaholism as a Syndrome. J Occup Health. 2006;11(1):52-62.

[75] Serrano-fernández MJ, Boada-grair J, Gil-ripolp C, Vigil-colet A. A predictive study of antecedent variables of workaholism. Psicothema 2016;28(4):401-7.

[76] McMillan LH, O'Driscoll MP. Workaholism and health: Implications for organizations. ournal Organ Chang Manag. 2004;17(5):509-19.

[77] Salmela-Aro K, Nurmi J-E. Employees' motivational orientation and well-being at work: A personoriented approach. ournal Organ Chang Manag. 2004;17(5):471-89.

[78] Salanova, M.; López-González, A.A.; Llorens, S.; del Líbano, M.; Vicente-Herrero, M.T.; Tomás-Salvá, M. Your work may be killing you! Workaholism, sleep problems and cardiovascular risk. Work Stress 2016, 30, 228-242

[79] Andreassen CS, Griffiths MD, Sinha R, Hetland J. The Relationships between Workaholism and Symptoms of Psychiatric Disorders : A Large- Scale Cross-Sectional Study. PLoS One. 2016;11(5):1-19

[80] Shimazu A, Schaufeli WB, Taris TW. How does workaholism affect worker health and performance? The mediating role of coping. Int J Behav Med. 2010;17(2):154-60.

[81] Shimazu A, Schaufeli WB. Is workaholism good or bad for employee well-being? The distinctiveness of workaholism and work engagement among Japanese employees. Ind Health. 2009;47(5):495-502

[82] Engelbrecht GJ,Beer LT De, Schaufeli WB the relationships between work intensity, workaholism, burnout, and self-reported musculoskeletal complaints.Human Factors and Ergonomics in Manufacturing &Service İndustries 2020 ; 30(1) : 59-70 https//doi.org/10.1002/hfm.2082

[83] Schaufeli WB, Bakker AB, Van der Heijden FMM., Prins JT. Workaholism Among Medical Residents : It Is the Combination of Working Excessively and Compulsively That Counts. Int J Stress Manag. 2009;16(4):249-72

[84] Pallesen S, Mitsem M, Kvale G, Johnsen B, Molde H. Outcome of psychological treatments of pathological gambling: A review and meta-analysis. Addiction. 2005;100(10):1412-22

[85] Lundahl BW, Kunz C, Brownell C, Tollefson D, Burke BL. A meta-analysis of Motivational Interviewing: Twenty-five years of empirical studies. Res Soc Work Pract. 2010;20(2):137-60

[86] Burwell R, Chen CP. The long work hours culture Causes, consequences and choices. In: Burke RJ, Cooper CL, editors. Positive psychology for work-life balance: A new approach in treating workaholism. Lancaster, UK: Emeral Group Publishing Limited; 2008. p. 295-313

[87] Fry LW, Matherly LL, Vitucci S. Spiritual leadership theory as a source for future theory, research, and recovery from workaholism. In: Burke RJ, editor. Research companion to working time and work addiction. Cheltenham, UK: Edward Elgar; 2006. p. 330-52

Chapter 13

Influence of Tunisian Revolution on Bullying at Work in Interns and Residents

Irtyah Merchaoui, Ines Rassas, Marouen Hayouni, Nidhal Mlik, Feten Mhenni, Imen Miled and Charfeddine Amri

Abstract

This study aims to compare prevalence and determinants of workplace bullying, in interns and residents before and after Tunisian revolution and to assess its influence on their quality of life. It was a two-step-cross-sectional study, carried out in 2009 and in 2016, in547 interns and residents in 2009 and 667 in 2016.The prevalence of workplace bullying decreased significantly ($p < 10^{-3}$) between 2009 (74%) and 2016 (43.6%). It was related to the professional status, gender, seniority, deliberate choice of medicine, satisfaction, serious family problems and hobbies in 2009 while it was related to professional status, nature of specialty, deliberate choice of medical studies and the satisfaction of the practice of Medicine in 2016. Most common acts were similar between both cohorts. Median mental and physical quality of life scores were below the mean baseline scores in both cohorts with no significant difference. Despite decrease in workplace bullying rate between both cohorts, its perception has not changed. Lawful criminalization, raising public awareness to reduce this phenomenon and prevent its negative effects are preventive measures to apply.

Keywords: bullying, quality of life, internship and residency, social changes

1. Introduction

The socio-cultural changes in the modern world as well as the changes in the mediatization contributed to the emergence of the notion of moral harassment at work (MHW). Research about workplace bullying has continued to grow since Scandinavian investigations about school bullying emerged in the late 70s.

Workplace bullying is "a situation in which one or more persons are systematically and over a long period, targeted by repeated, health-harming mistreatment by one or more perpetrators. Person(s) exposed to the mistreatment has (have) difficulty in defending themselves against this treatment" [1]. This is a complex and dynamic notion that is not the subject of a consensual definition despite the growing scientific interest [1–4].

Insidious violence and hostile actions can be grouped in four categories: isolation and refusal of communication, humiliating attitudes or disqualifying remarks in order to offend human dignity, intimidations aiming at terrorizing the targeted person so that it leads to submission or leave [1].

Health care professionals are highly exposed to MHW and facing the pain and death of patients [5, 6]. Young doctors, interns and residents, are besides obliged to follow a highly demanding apprenticeship. In fact, they live in a state of chronic stress and are subjected to significant mental burden facing the challenge to learn, to work in a team, to become competent, responsible and empathic physicians and at the same time to provide medical services although the hostile atmosphere and in often unfavorable conditions. This kind of heavy occupational atmosphere, promoting the development of MHW, has been highlighted by a previous study conducted in 2009 [7].

Tunisian jasmine revolution, initiated to face critical economic situation, frustration, hopelessness, injustice, corruption and political domination, conducted to a new approach of justice and dignity [8]. It was followed little by little, by the procession of freedom of expression that, sometimes exceeded rights limits.

Otherwise, hospitals' working conditions, within the after revolution, have significantly worsened, due to family patients' violence and lack of equipment, leading to heavy work conditions affecting the medical practice of young doctors and doubly exposing them to harassment at work.

The aims of the study were to:

- Compare the prevalence and the perception of workplace bullying in interns and residents before and after revolution.

- Assess the influence of workplace bullying on their quality of life.

2. Methods

2.1 Study design and participants

This is a comparative cross-sectional study, practiced in two stages: 2009 and 2016.The cohort of participants included all interns and medical residents practicing within the teaching hospitals attached to the Faculty of Medicine of Monastir-Tunisia. This current study was based on data of 547 Participants in 2009 and 667 ones in 2016.It took place during approximately the same period in both stages: October and November2009 and then in October, November and December 2016. Incomplete forms were not included in the study and no participant was excluded. Moreover, even though both studies have been performed in the same places, no overlap between both cohorts was noticed, because 2009 cohort, whether interns or residents, have already finish their curriculum in 2016. Finally, the study was approved by the regional ethical committee.

2.2 Measurements

2.2.1 Data collection

Data on MHW were obtained through the administration of the same anonymous self-administered questionnaire distributed to the target population of 2009 and 2016.A unique investigator distributed the self-questionnaire to all the cohort of interns and residents in hospital departments. He guaranteed to each participant the anonymity and asked him/her to respond as sincerely as possible and trust his immediate reaction rather than a long thoughtful answer.

2.2.2 Outcome variables

a. Socio-professional data: gathering

- Socio-demographic characteristics: age, gender, marital status.
- Occupational characteristics: the professional status, the nature of specialty and seniority at work.
- Environmental characteristics such as number of children, distance between the residence and the workplace, means of transport, heavy family problems, hobbies and sports activities, work satisfaction.
- Alcohol-smoking habits

b. Workplace bullying:

It was assessed through the Negative Acts Questionnaire Revised or NAQ-R, which is a standardized self-questionnaire, made of 22 items. None of them is directly referring to harassment. Many practical and scientific studies have concluded to its validity and reliability on evaluating this phenomenon. It has also been validated in several countries of the world as a standardized instrument for assessment of moral harassment at work [9–11].

Each kind of behavior is increasingly leveled from 1 to 5 depending on the repetition of this act in the last six months: never, sometimes, once a month, once a week, and daily.

Negative acts mentioned were gathered in two types of behaviors: People-related behaviors and Work-related behaviors.

A person is considered to be a victim of psychological harassment if he or she has been suffering of any of these acts at least once per week in the last six months.

This self-questionnaire also helps to identify the most widespread negative act in a workplace.

At the end of this self-questionnaire, there is a 23rd question preceded by a definition of "mobbing" at work. It is interested in harassment at work as generally perceived by the person. The term harassment has been replaced by the term "mobbing at work".

Mobbing at work was defined as "a situation where one or more people perceive themselves as the target of negative acts from one or more people over a long period of time and have difficulties in defending themselves against these people (a single incident is not regarded as "mobbing").

We chose to use the NAQ-R score as a dependent continuous variable.

c. The Quality of Life Impact:

The SF8 'health survey' scale is a standardized and valid self-questionnaire that explores health and well-being of persons [12, 13]. We got the license of the Quality Metric Office of Grants and Scholarly Research, number QM038831 [14].

It contains eight questions exploring the following dimensions: Health as perceived by the subject, repercussion of physical health on daily activities, pain, physical activity, vitality, social activity, psychic health, repercussions of mental health on daily activities.

It allows to calculate two scores using a specialized software: the overall physical score (PCS: physical component score), which is the average of the first four sections; and the overall mental score (MCS: Mental component score) which is the average of the last four items.

These two scores range from 0 (the worst health state) to 100 (the more favorable state of health). The score 50 represents the average score or the standard of American population.

2.3 The statistical study

The results were analyzed with the SPSS software version 21. The univariate comparative study was conducted using cross-tabulations with the chi-square test for comparison of discontinuous variables and T-student test to establish the difference in averages between both populations. Verification of the normality of both quantitative variables PCS and MCS was made. The threshold of significance has been set at 0.05.

Multi-varied analysis was performed using binary logistic regression multi-varied step-by-step to identify variables that are related significantly to harassment at work, regardless of the other variables respectively in 2009 and 2016, with a risk taken at 0.05. The criterion for including independent variables in the regression model was a threshold of significance <0.2.

Results of both cohorts were presented in chronological order (2009/2016).

3. Results

3.1 Descriptive and comparative study of socio-professional and demographic data of both cohorts

In 2009, the study was conducted among 547 participants (218 interns and 113 residents) working in Monastir and Mahdia teaching hospitals with a total response rate of 60.5%. In 2016, the study was conducted among 667 participants (215 interns and 120 residents) in the same teaching hospitals with a global response rate of 50.22%. No significant statistical difference in response rates was noticed between both stages of the study.

The respective specific response rates scheduled according to the chronological progress of the study showed that the interns response rates were about 62.8% in 2009 and 58.74% in 2016 while residents ones were respectively 50.1% and 39.86%.

3.1.1 Socio-demographic and occupational characteristics

Both populations were statistically comparable in all their sociodemographic and occupational characteristics in both cohorts.

In addition, the participation rates of interns were higher than those of residents (62.8%/62.1%) and the majority of people interviewed were working in medical services in both cohorts (**Table 1**).

3.1.2 Environmental characteristics

a. Family characteristics

Most of participants had no children in 2009 and 2016 Cohorts (90.9%/87.5%). However, 2016 interns and residents were significantly more plaintive about serious family problems ($p < 10^{-3}$) (**Table 1**).

Environmental characteristics		2009 Cohort	2016 cohort	P
Professional status (%)	Interns	65.9	64.2	NS
	Residents	34.12	35.8	
Specialty (%)	Medical	62.8	62.1	0.04
	Surgical	35.4	37.9	
	Fundamental	1.8	0	NS
Children Number: (N)	0	90.9	87.5	
	1	9.1	12.5	<10.3
Serious Families Problems: (%)	yes	11.2	46.6	
	No	88.8	53.4	NS
Means of transport: (%)	On foot	30.9	31.9	
	bicycle	3.9	0.9	
	car	32.6	31.6	
	Public transport	32.6	35.6	<10.3
Leisure activities: (%)	Never	42	46.5	
	Rarely	48	33.5	
	Always	10	20	NS
Smoking: (%)	Yes	22.7	17.9	
	No	77.3	82.1	NS
Alcohol:	Yes	13.9	13.1	
	No	86.1	86.9	
Career choice	Yes	78.9	85.4	0.018
	No	21.1	14.6	
Practice expectation satisfaction:	Yes	41.4	41.8	NS
	No	58.6	58.2	

Table 1.
Distribution of both cohorts according to environmental and occupational characteristics.

b. Accessibility to workplace

The daily average distance to attend workplace was statistically higher in 2016 cohort ($p = 0.012$).

All means of transport (moving on foot, by car and public transport) were equivalently used in both cohorts ($p = 0.075$) (**Table 1**).

c. Sports activities and hobbies:

On one hand, participants in both cohorts complained about the lack of time to practice leisure activities (90%; 80%). On the other hand, the leisure activity practicing rate has significantly doubled, between 2009 (10%) and 2016 (20%). ($p < 10^{-3}$) (**Table 1**).

d. Alcohol-smoking habits

Both study cohorts showed no significant difference neither in smoking habit ($p = 0.07$) nor in alcohol consumption ($p = 0.43$) (**Table 1**).

e. Satisfaction with the choice of medical curriculum and expectations of the practice of Medicine

The rate of students who deliberately chose to lead a medical career has significantly increased between 2009 (78.9%) and 2016 (85.4%) ($p = 0.01$).

However, there was no significant difference between both cohorts in satisfaction with medical practicing expectations (**Table 1**).

3.2 Analytical study of the determinants of workplace bullying in both cohorts

3.2.1 Univariate analysis of 2009 cohort

Workplace bullying was significantly linked to younger age ($p = <10^{-3}$), occupational status of intern ($p = <10^{-3}$), surgical specialties ($p = 0.046$), shorter seniority at work ($p = 0.003$), serious family problems ($p = 0.001$), as well as to disappointing medical practice ($p < 10^{-3}$).

All the remaining socio-demographic, occupational or environmental features had no significant relationship with bullying at work in interns and residents in 2009 (**Table 2**).

Characteristics	**2009 cohort**			**2016 cohort**		
	p	OR	$IC_{95\%}$	p	OR	$IC_{95\%}$
Age (Younger)	$< 10^{-3}$			0.00		
Gender (Female)	0.08			NS		
Marital status	NS					
Occupational Status	$< 10^{-3}$	0.3	[0.1–0.5]	NS	0.3	[0.24–0.6]
(Interm)				$< 10^{-3}$		
Specialty (Surgery)	0.04	0.14	[0.03–0.6]		1.7	[1.1–2.7]
Seniority (Shorter)	0.00			0.016		
Children (N)	NS			0.004		
Serious Family	0.00			NS		
Problems	NS			NS		
Distance to work(km)	0.05			NS		
Public Means of	0.17			NS		
transport	NS			NS		
Leisure activities	NS			NS		
No Smoking	NS			NS		
No Alcohol	NS					
Medical curriculum	**NS**					
choice						
Medical practice	< **10-3**	2.5	[1.52–4.16]	< **10-3**		
Satisfaction				< **10-3**		

Table 2.
Univariate analysis of determinants of work bullying in both cohorts.

3.2.2 Multivariate analysis of 2009 cohort

After binary logistic regression, the determinant model influencing the advent of MHW was made of intern job position ($p < 10^{-3}$), female gender ($p < 10^{-3}$), shorter seniority ($p = 0.02$), the deliberate choice of medical career ($p < 10^{-3}$), dissatisfaction with medical practice ($p < 10^{-3}$), serious family problems ($p < 10^{-3}$) and lack of leisure activities ($p = 0.01$) (**Table 3**).

3.2.3 Univariate analysis of 2016 cohort

In 2016, workplace bullying was significantly related to younger age ($p = 0.003$), to the internship status ($p = <10^{-3}$), to surgical specialties ($p = 0.046$), to a shorter seniority at work ($p = 0.004$), to the use of public transport ($p = 0.016$), to compulsory choice of medical curriculum ($p < 10^{-3}$) as well as to disappointing medical practice ($p < 10^{-3}$) (**Table 2**).

All the remaining socio-demographic, occupational or environmental features had no significant relationship with bullying at work in interns and residents in 2016.

3.2.4 Multivariate analysis of 2016 cohort

The binary logistic regression showed an explanatory model of the moral harassment at work for 2016 Cohort consisting of job position ($p = 0.008$), specialty ($p = 0.031$), deliberate choice of medical studies ($p < 10^{-3}$) and Medical practice dissatisfaction ($p < 10^{-3}$) (**Table 4**).

3.2.5 Comparison of both cohorts' scores

Comparison of the NAQ-R scores between 2009 and 2016 showed that it was significantly higher in 2009 score, while no difference was noticed in bullying scores between both cohorts (**Table 5**).

Determinants	**P**
Job Position (Intern)	<10–3
Gender (Female)	0.001
Seniority (Shorter)	0.023
Choice (Compulsory)	0.006
Medical Practice (Disappointing)	0.002
Family Problems (Serious)	0.007
Leisure Activities (Lack)	0.011

Table 3.
Multivariate model of moral harassment at work in 2009 cohort.

Determinants	**p**
Job position (intern)	0.008
Specialty (Surgery)	0.031
Choice (Compulsory)	< 10–3
Medical Practice (Disappointing)	< 10–3

Table 4.
Multivariate model explaining workplace bullying in 2016 cohort.

NAQ results		2009 Cohort		2016 cohort		p
		N	%	N	%	
NAQ-R	Harassed	245	74	146	43.6	<10–3
	Not harassed	86	26	189	56.4	
Mobbing	Yes	23	6.9	17	5.1	0.19
	No	308	93.1	318	94.9	

Table 5.
Comparison of both cohorts' NAQ-R scores.

3.3 Impact of MHW on the quality of life

3.3.1 Mental health score (MCS)

The median MCS was 40.3 ± 12 in 2009 and 40.61 ± 13.48 in 2016. No significant difference was recorded for the MCS. However, the majority of respondents had a mental health score below the standard of 50 in 2009 Cohort (86.1%) as well in 2016 Cohort (84.8%).

Univariate regression showed that workplace bullying influenced the mental quality of mental life significantly in 2009 ($p < 10^{-3}$, SD = [2.63; 7.06]) as well as in 2016 ($p < 10^{-3}$, SD = [3.14, 7.04]).

3.3.2 Physical health score (PCS)

The median score for the PSC was 45.6- ± 11.72009 and 45.36 ± 11.09 in 2016 with no statistically significant difference between both cohorts.

In 2009 Cohort as well as in 2016 one, the majority of participants had comparable PSC < 50 (69.8%/72%) with no significant difference.

Univariate regression showed that workplace bullying had significantly influenced the physical quality of life in 2009 (p = 0.013, SD = [0.49; 4.2]) and in 2016 (p = 0.004, SD = [0.86, 4.37]).

4. Discussion

The present survey showed that, according to the objective criteria of NAQ-R, prevalence of bullying at work in interns and residents attached to the faculty of Medicine of Monastir has significantly decreased between 2009 and 2016. However, according to the last item if NAQ-R about subjective criteria, the rate perception of workplace bullying was similar in 2009 and 2016, consequently, in both cohorts, young doctors do not seem to recognize themselves as victims of moral harassment.

As for the quality of life, no significant differences were found, between both cohorts concerning the mental and physical plans. However, both populations medians were below the American standard of 50 and participants' scores of mental and physical qualities of life have been significantly altered because of MHW in both cohorts.

The concept of moral harassment was gradually introduced in mid-80s by Norwegian and Swedish occupational psychologists such as Leymann and Einarsen [3, 15].

The presence of certain characteristics or criteria is required by the most researchers such as the persistence of negative acts (for at least six months), repetition (for example at least once a week) and notion of "Imbalance of power" between the generator of harassment and the victim. Moreover, several authors have also incorporated into their definitions the adverse effects of this phenomenon on victims, including psychological effects [2, 3, 10, 16–20].

As for Mobbing, it has been defined by Leymann [21] as a process of harassment of a victim by one or more persecutors as a result of ordinary conflict. This is a repeated process over a long period based on words, gestures, writings, of such a nature as to affect the personality, dignity or the physical or psychic integrity of the other.

In the present survey, we have opted for the adoption of the same measurement tool (NAQ-R) and the same definition of MHW for both cohorts, but despite this comparability, our survey showed that prevalence of bullying at work in interns and residents has significantly decreased between 2009 and 2016.

2011's Tunisian revolution, with the accompanying socio-cultural changes, such as freedom of expression procession, the creation of the Tunisian Association of Young doctors, a representative union organization of interns and residents founded in December 2016, the media coverage of violence against interns and residents on social networks, seem to be responsible, at least in a part, for this decline in the prevalence of MHW.

The same phenomenon has been observed other where, such as Europe, where the prevalence of MHW decreased from 30% in 2003 to 15% in 2011 [2, 22].

Despite the cultural and social evolution, moral harassment at work is still unknown in Tunisia, and up to now, there are no laws incriminating this phenomenon.

In the literature, studies carried out among health personnel based on the NAQ-R, report figures ranging from 8 to 32% [23–30].

Physicians are at a high risk of workplace bullying. Indeed, they are in direct contact with the patients, with their pain, suffering and death, with their parents and families, and they assume all legal responsibility in case of safety care incident [5, 6].

Furthermore, Medicine is a very hierarchical profession where medical trainees, interns and residents are at the bottom of curriculum and represent the basis of patients' medical care especially in university hospitals. They are, therefore, more exposed to different types of negative behaviors and bullying.

Taking into account, the lack of staff, the lack of equipment,the lack of autonomy, the lack of teamwork, support and feedback and the dependence on seniors' opinions, it is easy understandable that all these factors of stress and frustration lead to the emergence of different negative acts of MHW [31, 32] . This can explain the high prevalence of bullying at work among young doctors and medical students in comparison with the general population and other health professions [33].

The present study showed that the most widespread negative acts were identical between both cohorts of 2009 and 2016.

However, some negative acts such as switching key activities by tasks below the skills and by mundane or unpleasant activities have significantly increased in 2016 while others have significantly decreased, such as putting pressure on young doctors not to claim their rights like vacations, maternity and sick leave.

Since 2011, Tunisian country has been facing many socio-economic problems [34]. In fact, teaching hospitals are concerned with an increasing deterioration of work conditions especially perceived by young doctors. The lack of autonomy, the progressive installation of a culture of mediocrity lead, on one hand, to the proliferation of the private sector at the expense of the public one, and to a mass brain drain of Tunisian medical skills to foreign countries on the other hand; these factors had bad consequences on our health care system [35].

Nevertheless, even in countries where socio-economic stability is the rule, dissatisfaction with the work conditions is reported [36].

The insufficient number of doctors and staff to deal with growing number of patients and a growing demand for care, has been reported as the origin of MHW among nurses in Japan [23], South Korea [28], the United Kingdom [24] and violence in hospitals in India [37].

Excessive supervision of work was another type of negative acts, frequently reported by interns and residents in both cohorts. It was also one of the most reported negative acts by young doctors in the United States in 2015 (44%) [38].

The socio-cultural changes, arising after Tunisian revolution, allowed young people to challenge some department heads' unfair decisions and to claim their rights [39].

Besides, the negative act relating to the deliberate ignorance of opinions or points of view were common among trainee physicians [40–42] as well as among healthcare givers [43]. Such inappropriate behavior can interfere with the relationship and create a hostile environment that can negatively influence work.

A meta-analysis published in 2014, 51 studies about MHW and discrimination in medical trainees [44] has shown that the most common negative act was verbal abuse (3–28%) and racial and gender discrimination (4–19%).The same respective types of discrimination, in addition to religious one, were reported in medical students in Saudi Arabia [45].

Contrary to our study, several other studies conducted among practicing physicians and those in the process of training showed, that verbal abuse was a widespread behavior [33, 38, 42, 45–49]. This type of act could lead to depressive symptoms among medical students [50].

Even though it was rare in the present study, humiliation is a negative act of MHW and has been found to be common in multiple studies conducted among physicians in training courses and health personnel [24, 38, 41, 51–54] .

Moreover, physical violence in hospitals was the least negative act reported in some harassment investigations among young doctors [40, 44, 48] and it did not significantly increase between 2009 and 2016 in our study.

As for the perception of workplace bullying in the present study, young doctors in both cohorts, do not seem to recognize themselves as victims of moral harassment whereas the prevalence of perceived MHW in the literature is varying from 27–52% [38, 47, 55–57].

It seems that, humiliation and offense resulting from the recognition of themselves as harassed, refer to a lower position, weakness and passivity leading to the deny of MHW by victims. Besides, victims of harassment do not want to be confronted with this truth thinking that it is their own fault [58] or that of the organization in which they work and rather than stalker's one [59]. Others believe that recognizing victim status especially during their temporary internships will call their professional future into question [46, 60, 61].

As for identified determinants of moral harassment at work in our study, the job position of intern, the deliberate choice of medical studies and the dissatisfaction with the medical practice were the common determinants in both cohorts.

Serious family problems, seniority and the lack of leisure time were also apart from the explanatory model of 2009, while the nature of specialty was an additional determinant in 2016.

Generally, young age is correlated with MHW among medical trainees because of their vulnerability to stress and their sensitivity to criticism [62].

Female gender was not a determinant of harassment in both studies, but it persisted after multiple logistic regression in 2009. It would seem therefore, that gender discrimination among young doctors decreased after the socio-cultural changes of the last 8 years.

In the literature, women in the general work field, with their tendency to vulnerability, are the most exposed to harassment [24, 26, 38, 41, 63, 64] unlike men who are predominant in management positions and consequently mostly stalkers [16, 47, 65].

In addition, in the medical sector, women face many difficulties to reconcile professional and private life [66].

Dealing with the occupational determinants, in our study, a lower seniority was a predisposing factor to the MHW in 2009. The youngest doctors are those with shortest seniority and therefore the most vulnerable to MHW.

Being intern, as young trainee, was also a risk factor for bullying in both cohorts. In fact, interns are located at the bottom of the medical professional hierarchy, and are consequently exposed to a high level of stress because of a low autonomy and a high level of requirement. Thus, interns are more predisposed to workplace bullying [31, 41, 62].

On another side, surgical specialty was a determining factor of bullying in 2016 cohort while it appears to have been a confounding factor in the 2009 Cohort.

Surgery is a specialty that requires strength and toughness, which leads to some negative acts of harassment and explain our results.

In the literature, some specialties with heavy workload and ubiquitous stress predispose more than others to MHW in the healthcare givers. Gynecological obstetrics specialty has been predictive of a high rate of MHW among residents in Mexico [67].

Finally, verbal aggression among doctors in the United States has been more important in the specialties of interventional radiology and in general surgery unlike pediatrics [48].

Regarding the dissatisfaction with the work practice, it was significantly related to moral harassment score according to NAQ-R in both cohorts. Job satisfaction, as it has been defined by Locke [68], is an affective and emotional response of a person in face of a work situation resulting from the match between what the person wants (his expectations) and what he/she gets out of his/her job. Thus, dissatisfaction can contribute to emotional exhaustion, mental and physical weariness of professionals and then the desire to leave the profession [49, 68, 69].

In the literature some determinants are probably risk factors for harassment. Indeed, some changes in workplace such as diversification, staff management changes, downsizing, salary reductions or increasing working time and even the dimensions of locals can cause conflicts and influence negatively on the job which can explain the high level of MHW in a hospital [27, 70, 71].

In addition, several organizational determinants influence considerably the level of harassment in these environments, such as management of work (too authoritarian or too passive), conditions (insecurity at work) and work dynamics (workload, cognitive demand, abuse of power, interpersonal conflict), the constraints of time and cultural norms (commoditization of the bullying as a Performance tool) within a workplace [72, 73].

In Tunisia, the new democratic transition has contributed to the emergence of violence in the country following the appearance of religious extremists' groups, the accentuation forms of racial and sexual discrimination and violence in some protests against the government [74]. So, the mediatization of the incredible increase of violence against hospital doctors since 2011 in Tunisia could be also factors contributing to and trivialize harassment in hospitals.

The compulsory choice of Medical curriculum was another determinant factor in genesis of MHW among young doctors after logistic regression both in 2009 and 2016.

Young doctors whose medical career was not initiated by a personal choice were unhappy and frustrated with their studies and more exposed to the harassment because they are more vulnerable to negative acts.

On the other side, the satisfaction of choosing a medical career has significantly increased in 2016 compared to 2009.This could be explained a wider autonomy in the career choices for Tunisian bachelors since 2011, and by broadening the residency prospects of trainees, in fact residency positions have almost doubled since 2009.

As for the impact of bullying on participants' quality of life, it significantly influenced the quality of mental life regardless of the study cohort, but no significant difference was found between 2009 and 2016 and most of scores were below the standard average of 50.

Despite the decline in the rate of MHW in 2016, the quality of mental life did not change after the revolution. This may be related to other factors than the MHW upon which social or managerial factors, working conditions, work-family interface quality, social support, marital status and income ... [75, 76].

In the latest study conducted by 'Word Happiness' in 2017 regarding the satisfaction of life and happiness based on certain criteria such as health, social support, freedom and corruption, Tunisia was among the lowest ranked countries (rank of 102 out of 155 countries) [77].

The alteration of interns and resident mental quality of life can be also attributed to the fact that the internship is a period of chronic stress for young doctors who face the challenge of learning to work as a team, to become competent, responsible and empathic doctors and at the same time ensuring the best medical benefits in a sometimes competitive and even hostile climate.

The influence of MHW on the mental quality of life has been demonstrated in literature both in the general population [77, 78] and in the health caregivers [78, 79] and some authors assert that mental disorders are also predictors of harassment [79–81].

If we consider, the influence of MHW on the quality of physical life, the latter significantly altered the physical quality of life in both cohorts without significant difference between them and scores were below the American standard of 50.

In the literature, MHW has deleterious effects on physical health. It increased cardiovascular risk and caused musculoskeletal pain in addition to other medical problems [62, 73].

The new scheme of residency ship, consisting in pending months from June to December with long periods of preparation, leads to inactivity, and spending most of the day on screen and desk could explain the lack of improvement in the quality of physical life despite the significant increase in leisure time and the regression of the MHW in 2016 comparatively to 2009.

Considering the limits of our study, despite the decrease in the participation rate in 2016, the sample of the studied population remains representative of the general population. Some factors could influence the participation rate in both cohorts: some of the interns and residents were unmotivated, others could not answer our questionnaire due to lack of time and excessive workload. Many of them also found that the questionnaire was too long. The lower participation rate of residents compared to interns' one can be explained by their heavier workloads. Finally, the abstention of some participants can also be explained by the perception of MHW as a taboo subject or lack of conviction of the usefulness of such investigations.

The rate of participation in workplace bullying investigations among young physicians in literature varied between 22.1 and 72% [40, 41, 55, 63, 82].

Regarding the used tools, the NAQ and the SF8 are both validated and frequently used in different professional sectors and in various languages. But, due to the absence of a validated version in Tunisian dialect or in Arabic, we opted for the use of the French validated version which is commonly understandable by our study population because all medical studies are performed in French in Tunisia.

However, the disadvantage of the NAQ-R is that it asks a direct question at the end, about the self-perception of moral harassment. The respondents tend to deny this suffering, either out of shame or lack of motivation or unconscious denial of reality. This could be the cause of underestimation of results.

As for the quality of life, the SF8 provides a simple method for evaluating general mental and physical health; it has the advantage to be a brief and a valid questionnaire.

5. Conclusion

Health care professions, especially in young doctors, are at high-risk of moral harassment, due to required interactions with patients and their parents, requested performance of learning and the advent of violence against healthcare professionals after Tunisian revolution. The present study showed that MHW had significantly decreased in2016 according to the objective assessment by NAQ-R score. No significant difference between both cohorts perception of MHW was shown which can be explained by the lack of awareness of this phenomenon and by the absence of Tunisian legislation against harassment.

The determinants of the MHW in 2009 were the job position, gender, and seniority, choice of medicine satisfaction, serious family problems and leisure activities; while in 2016, they were the job position, the specialty nature, the choice of medical studies and the satisfaction of the exercise of Medicine. Finally, MHW negatively influenced the quality of mental and physical life in a comparable way in the two steps of investigation.

The promulgation of a law penalizing the MHW has become urgent especially after the revisions of the post revolution law texts. Politicians should focus on this major issue because MHW has many bad effects on the personal, social and organizational level. It is also important to set up training and awareness programs about MHW to prevent its emergence and reduce its deleterious effects.

Author details

Irtyah Merchaoui*, Ines Rassas, Marouen Hayouni, Nidhal Mlik, Feten Mhenni, Imen Miled and Charfeddine Amri
Department of Occupational Health and Ergonomics, Faculty of Medicine of Monastir, University of Monastir, Monastir, Tunisia

*Address all correspondence to: irtyah@gmail.com

References

[1] Hirigoyen M-F. Le harcèlement moral, un symptôme de la société moderne. Ann Méd-Psychol Rev Psychiatr. 2016 Sep;174(7):575-9.

[2] Branch S, Ramsay S, Barker M. Workplace Bullying, Mobbing and General Harassment: A Review: Workplace Bullying: A Review. Int J Manag Rev. 2013 Jul;15(3):280-99.

[3] Karabulut AT. Bullying: Harmful and Hidden Behavior in Organizations. Procedia - Soc Behav Sci. 2016 Aug;229:4-11.

[4] Saunders P, Huynh A, Goodman-Delahunty J. Defining workplace bullying behaviour professional lay definitions of workplace bullying. Int J Law Psychiatry. 2007 Jul;30(4-5):340-54.

[5] Méchin O. Effets sur les soignants de la douleur et de la souffrance des patients. Médecine Palliat Soins Support - Accompagnement - Éthique. 2013 Aug;12(4):201-6.

[6] Gheorghiev C, Gault C. Risques psycho-sociaux à l'hôpital : illustrations cliniques et réflexions autour de la place d'un idéal de soin chez les soignants. Ann Méd-Psychol Rev Psychiatr. 2016 Jun;174(5):393-6.

[7] Mhenni F. Etude de la souffrance mentale au travail chez les stagiaires internés et résidentsenmédecine.

[8] Hibou B, editor. La Tunisie en révolution? Paris: Éd. Karthala; 2011. 172 p. (Politique africaine).

[9] Petrović IB, Vukelić M, Čizmić S. Rocking at 81 and Rolling at 34: ROC Cut-Off Scores for the Negative Acts Questionnaire–Revised in Serbia. Front Psychol [Internet]. 2017 Jan 9 [cited 2020 Jun 24];7. Available from: http://journal.frontiersin.org/article/10.3389/fpsyg.2016.02058/full

[10] Cowie H, Naylor P, Rivers I, Smith PK, Pereira B. Measuring workplace bullying. Aggress Violent Behav. 2002 Jan;7(1):33-51.

[11] Einarsen S, Hoel H, Notelaers G. Measuring exposure to bullying and harassment at work: Validity, factor structure and psychometric properties of the Negative Acts Questionnaire-Revised. Work Stress. 2009 Jan;23(1):24-44.

[12] Roberts B, Browne J, Ocaka K, Oyok T, Sondorp E. The reliability and validity of the SF-8 with a conflict-affected population in northern Uganda. Health Qual Life Outcomes. 2008;6(1):108.

[13] Tokuda Y, Okubo T, Ohde S, Jacobs J, Takahashi O, Omata F, et al. Assessing Items on the SF-8 Japanese Version for Health-Related Quality of Life: A Psychometric Analysis Based on the Nominal Categories Model of Item Response Theory. Value Health. 2009 Jun;12(4):568-73.

[14] SF Health Surveys.

[15] Agervold M. Bullying at work: A discussion of definitions and prevalence, based on an empirical study. Scand J Psychol. 2007 Apr;48(2):161-72.

[16] Samnani A-K, Singh P. 20 Years of workplace bullying research: A review of the antecedents and consequences of bullying in the workplace. Aggress Violent Behav. 2012 Nov;17(6):581-9.

[17] Volk AA, Dane AV, Marini ZA. What is bullying? A theoretical redefinition. Dev Rev. 2014 Dec;34(4):327-43.

[18] Chirilă T, Constantin T. Understanding Workplace Bullying Phenomenon through its Concepts: A Literature Review. Procedia - Soc Behav Sci. 2013 Jul;84:1175-9.

[19] Swearer SM, Hymel S. Understanding the psychology of bullying: Moving toward a social-ecological diathesis–stress model. Am Psychol. 2015;70(4):344-53.

[20] Becton JB, Gilstrap JB, Forsyth M. Preventing and correcting workplace harassment: Guidelines for employers. Bus Horiz. 2017 Jan;60(1):101-11.

[21] Masclet G. Pour optimiser le soin, il faut donner du sens au travail. Psychol Trav Organ. 2010;16(4):391-412.

[22] Lipscomb J, London M, McPhaul KM, Ghaziri ME, Lydecker A, Geiger-Brown J, et al. The Prevalence of Coworker Conflict Including Bullying in a Unionized U.S. Public Sector Workforce. Violence Vict. 2015;30(5):813-29.

[23] Yokoyama M, Suzuki M, Takai Y, Igarashi A, Noguchi-Watanabe M, Yamamoto-Mitani N. Workplace bullying among nurses and their related factors in Japan: a cross-sectional survey. J Clin Nurs. 2016 Sep;25(17-18):2478-88.

[24] Carter M, Thompson N, Crampton P, Morrow G, Burford B, Gray C, et al. Workplace bullying in the UK NHS: a questionnaire and interview study on prevalence, impact and barriers to reporting. BMJ Open. 2013 Jun;3(6):e002628.

[25] Karatza C, Zyga S, Tziaferi S, Prezerakos P. Workplace Bullying Among the Nursing Staff of Greek Public Hospitals. Workplace Health Saf. 2017 Feb;65(2):57-64.

[26] Norton P, Costa V, Teixeira J, Azevedo A, Roma-Torres A, Amaro J, et al. Prevalence and Determinants of Bullying Among Health Care Workers in Portugal. Workplace Health Saf. 2017 May;65(5):188-96.

[27] An Y, Kang J. Relationship between Organizational Culture and Workplace Bullying among Korean Nurses. Asian Nurs Res. 2016 Sep;10(3):234-9.

[28] Yun S, Kang J, Lee Y-O, Yi Y. Work Environment and Workplace Bullying among Korean Intensive Care Unit Nurses. Asian Nurs Res. 2014 Sep;8(3):219-25.

[29] Farrell GA, Shafiei T. Workplace aggression, including bullying in nursing and midwifery: A descriptive survey (the SWAB study). Int J Nurs Stud. 2012 Nov;49(11):1423-31.

[30] Vogelpohl DA, Rice SK, Edwards ME, Bork CE. New Graduate Nurses' Perception of the Workplace: Have They Experienced Bullying? J Prof Nurs. 2013 Nov;29(6):414-22.

[31] Galam É, Multon R. Désaccords entre internes de médecine générale et seniors sur les soins aux patients. Gestion et impacts sur le hidden curriculum. Étude qualitative de 37 situations en Île-de-France. Presse Médicale. 2016 Mar;45(3):e39-50.

[32] Mahmood T. Dealing with trainees in difficulty. Facts Views Vis ObGyn. 2012;4(1):18-23.

[33] Karim S, Duchcherer M. Intimidation and harassment in residency: a review of the literature and results of the 2012 Canadian Association of Interns and Residents National Survey. Can Med Educ J. 2014;5(1):e50-57.

[34] Tunisie Diagnostic-pays systématique [Internet]. Groupe de la banque mondiale; Available from: http://documents.worldbank.org/curated/en/687071467997282070/pdf/102298-FRENCH-SCD-P151647-PUBLIC-Box394833B-TUNISIA-SCD-publication.pdf

[35] Berhouma M. The Arab Spring in Tunisia: Urgent Plea for a Public Health System (R)Evolution. World Neurosurg. 2013 Sep;80(3-4):260-3.

[36] Ferrand J-F, Trichereau J, Verret C, Rondier J-P, Viance P, Migliani R. Perception des risques professionnels et psychosociaux au sein de l'ensemble hospitalier militaire parisien. Arch Mal Prof Environ. 2013 Feb;74(1):16-33.

[37] Ambesh P. Violence against doctors in the Indian subcontinent: A rising bane. Indian Heart J. 2016 Sep;68(5):749-50.

[38] Chadaga AR, Villines D, Krikorian A. Bullying in the American Graduate Medical Education System: A National Cross-Sectional Survey. Amaral LAN, editor. PLOS ONE. 2016 Mar 16;11(3):e0150246.

[39] Etat des lieuxdes droits humainsen Tunisie [Internet]. 2017. Available from: https://www.euromedrights.org/wp-content/uploads/2017/01/2017-01-16-EuroMed-Droits-Note-finale-en-vue-du-SCDH-2017.pdf

[40] Schlitzkus LL, Vogt KN, Sullivan ME, Schenarts KD. Workplace Bullying of General Surgery Residents by Nurses. J Surg Educ. 2014 Nov;71(6):e149-54.

[41] Ling M, Young CJ, Shepherd HL, Mak C, Saw RPM. Workplace Bullying in Surgery. World J Surg. 2016 Nov;40(11):2560-6.

[42] Nyhsen CM, Patel P, O'Connell JE. Bullying and harassment – Are junior doctors always the victims? Radiography. 2016 Nov;22(4):e264-8.

[43] Chipps E, Stelmaschuk S, Albert NM, Bernhard L, Holloman C. Workplace bullying in the OR: Results of a descriptive study. AORN J. 2013 Nov;98(5):479-93.

[44] Fnais N, Soobiah C, Chen MH, Lillie E, Perrier L, Tashkhandi M, et al. Harassment and discrimination in medical training: a systematic review and meta-analysis. Acad Med J Assoc Am Med Coll. 2014 May;89(5):817-27.

[45] Iftikhar R, Tawfiq R, Barabie S. Interns & amp; rsquo; perceived abuse during their undergraduate training at King Abdul Aziz University. Adv Med Educ Pract. 2014 May;159.

[46] Zafar W, Siddiqui E, Ejaz K, Shehzad MU, Khan UR, Jamali S, et al. Health care personnel and workplace violence in the emergency departments of a volatile metropolis: results from Karachi, Pakistan. J Emerg Med. 2013 Nov;45(5):761-72.

[47] Lazarus JL, Hosseini M, Kamangar F, Levien DH, Rowland PA, Kowdley GC, et al. Verbal Aggressiveness Among Physicians and Trainees. J Surg Educ. 2016 Jul;73(4):756-60.

[48] Al-Shafaee M, Al-Kaabi Y, Al-Farsi Y, White G, Al-Maniri A, Al-Sinawi H, et al. Pilot study on the prevalence of abuse and mistreatment during clinical internship: a cross-sectional study among first year residents in Oman. BMJ Open. 2013;3(2):e002076.

[49] Crutcher RA, Szafran O, Woloschuk W, Chatur F, Hansen C. Family medicine graduates' perceptions of intimidation, harassment, and discrimination during residency training. BMC Med Educ. 2011 Dec;11(1):88.

[50] Castaldelli-Maia JM, Martins SS, Bhugra D, Machado MP, Andrade AG de, Alexandrino-Silva C, et al. Does ragging play a role in medical student depression - cause or effect? J Affect Disord. 2012 Aug;139(3):291-7.

[51] Lazare A, Levy RS. Apologizing for Humiliations in Medical Practice. Chest. 2011 Apr;139(4):746-51.

[52] Pradhan A, Page-Ramsey S, Buery-Joyner SD, Craig LB, Dalrymple JL, Forstein DA, et al. Undergraduate obstetrics and gynecology medical education: why are we underrated and underappreciated? Am J Obstet Gynecol. 2016 Mar;214(3):345-7.

[53] Stone JP, Charette JH, McPhalen DF, Temple-Oberle C. Under the Knife: Medical Student Perceptions of Intimidation and Mistreatment. J Surg Educ. 2015 Jul;72(4):749-53.

[54] Imran N, Jawaid M, Haider II, Masood Z. Bullying of junior doctors in Pakistan: a cross-sectional survey. Singapore Med J. 2010 Jul;51(7):592-5.

[55] Quine L. Workplace bullying in junior doctors: questionnaire survey. BMJ. 2002 Apr 13;324(7342):878-9.

[56] Ahmer S, Yousafzai AW, Bhutto N, Alam S, Sarangzai AK, Iqbal A. Bullying of Medical Students in Pakistan: A Cross-Sectional Questionnaire Survey. Syed E, editor. PLoS ONE. 2008 Dec 8;3(12):e3889.

[57] Bairy K, Thirumalaikolundusubramanian P, Sivagnanam G, Saraswathi S, Sachidananda A, Shalini A. Bullying among trainee doctors in Southern India: A questionnaire study. J Postgrad Med. 2007;53(2):87.

[58] Porto Serantes N, Araña Suárez M. Myths about workplace violence, harassment and bullying. Int J Sociol Law. 2006 Dec;34(4):229-38.

[59] Kakarika M, González-Gómez HV, Dimitriades Z. That wasn't our deal: A psychological contract perspective on employee responses to bullying. J Vocat Behav. 2017 Jun;100:43-55.

[60] Whiteside D, Stubbs B, Soundy A. Physiotherapy students' experiences of bullying on clinical internships: a qualitative study. Physiotherapy. 2014 Mar;100(1):41-6.

[61] Babaria P, Abedin S, Berg D, Nunez-Smith M. "I'm too used to it": A longitudinal qualitative study of third year female medical students' experiences of gendered encounters in medical education. Soc Sci Med. 2012 Apr;74(7):1013-20.

[62] Parikh JR, Harolds JA, Bluth EI. Workplace Bullying in Radiology and Radiation Oncology. J Am Coll Radiol. 2017 Aug;14(8):1089-93.

[63] Paice E, Aitken M, Houghton A, Firth-Cozens J. Bullying among doctors in training: cross sectional questionnaire survey: Table 1. BMJ. 2004 Sep 18; 329(7467):658-9.

[64] Ogunsemi OO, Alebiosu OC, Shorunmu OT. A survey of perceived stress, intimidation, harassment and well-being of resident doctors in a Nigerian Teaching Hospital. Niger J Clin Pract. 2010 Jun;13(2):183-6.

[65] Kim YS, Boyce WT, Koh Y-J, Leventhal BL. Time Trends, Trajectories, and Demographic Predictors of Bullying: A Prospective Study in Korean Adolescents. J Adolesc Health. 2009 Oct;45(4):360-7.

[66] Straehley CJ, Longo P. Family issues affecting women in medicine, particularly women surgeons. Am J Surg. 2006 Nov;192(5):695-8.

[67] Ortiz-León S, Jaimes-Medrano AL, Tafoya-Ramos SA, Mujica-Amaya ML, Olmedo-CancholaVH,Carrasco-RojasJA. [Experiences of bullying in medical residents]. Cir Cir. 2014 Jun;82(3): 290-301.

[68] Poilpot-Rocaboy G, Notelaers G, Hauge LJ. Exposition au harcèlement psychologique au travail : Impact sur la satisfaction au travail, l'implication organisationnelle et l'intention de départ. Psychol Trav Organ. 2015;21(4):358-79.

[69] Estryn-Behar M, Duville N, Menini M-L, Le Foll S, Le Nézet O, Bocher R. Mots à maux... Expression de la souffrance chez les soignants en psychiatrie. Étude comparative en France et dans trois autres pays européens. Ann Méd-Psychol Rev Psychiatr. 2006 Nov;164(9):732-48.

[70] Denis M-A, Fort E, Massardier-Pilonchery A. Facteurs de risques psycho-sociaux des situations de souffrance au travail dans la population d'un établissement hospitalier. Arch Mal Prof Environ. 2014 Jun;75(3):322-3.

[71] Ghadi V, Mounic V. La qualité de vie au travail dans la certification des établissements de santé. Arch Mal Prof Environ. 2012 Jun;73(3):232-8.

[72] Van den Brande W, Baillien E, De Witte H, Vander Elst T, Godderis L. The role of work stressors, coping strategies and coping resources in the process of workplace bullying: A systematic review and development of a comprehensive model. Aggress Violent Behav. 2016 Jul;29:61-71.

[73] Qureshi MI, Rasli AMd, Zaman K. A New Trilogy to Understand the Relationship among Organizational Climate, Workplace Bullying and Employee Health. Arab Econ Bus J. 2014 Oct;9(2):133-46.

[74] Schraeder PJ. Tunisia's Jasmine Revolution & the Arab Spring: Implications for International Intervention. Orbis. 2012 Sep;56(4): 662-75.

[75] Joulain M, Coulombier G. Liens entre vécu au travail et bien-être subjectif des infirmier(ère)s : des effets réciproques. Psychol Trav Organ. 2016 Sep;22(3):205-15.

[76] Escribà-Ag V, Tenas-Burillo JM. Psychological well-being among hospital personnel: the role of family demands and psychosocial work environment. Int Arch Occup Environ Health [Internet]. 2004 Aug [cited 2020 Jun 24];77(6). Available from: http://link.springer.com/10.1007/s00420-004-0525-2

[77] Helliwell JF, Layard R, Sachs J. World happiness report 2017. New York, N.Y.: Sustainable Development Solutions Network; 2017.

[78] Wright W, Khatri N. Bullying among nursing staff: Relationship with psychological/behavioral responses of nurses and medical errors. Health Care Manage Rev. 2015;40(2):139-47.

[79] Wolf LA, Perhats C, Delao AM, Clark PR. Workplace aggression as cause and effect: Emergency nurses' experiences of working fatigued. Int Emerg Nurs. 2017 Jul;33:48-52.

[80] Hogh A, Hansen ÅM, Mikkelsen EG, Persson R. Exposure to negative acts at work, psychological stress reactions and physiological stress response. J Psychosom Res. 2012 Jul;73(1):47-52.

[81] Hogh A, Conway PM, Grynderup MB, Gullander M, Willert MV, Mikkelsen EG, et al. Negative Acts at Work as Potential Bullying Behavior and Depression: Examining the Direction of the Association in a 2-Year Follow-Up Study. J Occup Environ Med. 2016 Mar;58(3):e72-9.

[82] Kacem I, Kalboussi H, Ayoub N, Brahem A, Maoua M, Boughattas W, et al. Burn-out chez les jeunes médecins: étude réalisée dans la région de Sousse. Ann Méd-Psychol Rev Psychiatr. 2017 Apr;175(4):332-8.